OXFORD MEDICAL PUBLICATIONS

UNICOMPARTMENTAL ARTHROPLASTY WITH THE OXFORD KNEE

David Murray

John Goodfellow

John O'Connor

Chris Dodd

UNICOMPARTMENTAL ARTHROPLASTY WITH THE OXFORD KNEE

John Goodfellow

John O'Connor

Christopher Dodd

David Murray

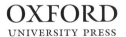

OXFORD

UNIVERSITY PRESS

OXFORD
UNIVERSITY PRESS

Great Clarendon Street, Oxford OX2 6DP

Oxford University Press is a department of the University of Oxford.
It furthers the University's objective of excellence in research, scholarship,
and education by publishing worldwide in

Oxford New York

Auckland Cape Town Dar es Salaam Hong Kong Karachi
Kuala Lumpur Madrid Melbourne Mexico City Nairobi
New Delhi Shanghai Taipei Toronto

With offices in

Argentina Austria Brazil Chile Czech Republic France Greece
Guatemala Hungary Italy Japan South Korea Poland Portugal
Singapore Switzerland Thailand Turkey Ukraine Vietnam

Oxford is a registered trade mark of Oxford University Press
in the UK and in certain other countries

Published in the United States
by Oxford University Press Inc., New York

A catalogue record for this title is available from the British Library

Library of Congress Cataloging in Publication Data

Unicompartmental arthroplasty with the Oxford Knee / John Goodfellow ... [et al.].
    p. ; cm.
 Includes bibliographical references and index.
 1. Arthroplasty. 2. Artificial knee.
 [DNLM: 1. Arthroplasty, Replacement, Knee–methods. 2. Knee Prosthesis. WE 870 U578 2006]
 1. Goodfellow, John.
 RD561.U55 2006
 617.5′820592–dc22   2006003817

Typeset by EXPO Holdings Sdn. Bhd., Malaysia

Printed in Great Britain

on acid-free paper by CPI Bath Press

ISBN 978–0–19–857–052–3 (Hbk) 0–19–857–052–X (HbK)

10 9 8 7 6 5 4 3 2 1

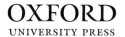

OXFORD
UNIVERSITY PRESS

Preface

A whole book, about one knee prosthesis! And only half a knee prosthesis at that!

The scope of this book is, actually, a little wider than the exclamations above suggest, but some excuse is surely required. We have written, in fact, about unicompartmental arthroplasty, an intellectually exciting and technically demanding subject for which the authors have a shared enthusiasm. However, since surgical expertise is gained slowly, most practitioners learn only one way of dealing with a particular clinical problem, and we are no exceptions. Our experience of treating unicompartmental arthritis over the last 25 years has been almost exclusively with our own invention, the Oxford Unicompartmental Knee, and we can only write with first-hand authority about that. We have, of course, tried to make good this deficiency from the published reports of other surgeons (whose experience, although different, is usually similarly limited); but, as with other history books, the realistic reader will expect only an *attempt* at a balanced view, and not necessarily an unbiased attempt.

Until very recently, unicompartmental arthroplasty itself was something of a niche activity. Most orthopaedic surgeons in the world did not use the method at all, and even its champions thought it appropriate for no more than a small proportion of arthritic knees in need of surgery. As will appear, we believe that as many as one-third of those who currently undergo total knee replacement may be better treated by unicompartmental arthroplasty. Soon, a million total knee arthroplasties will be performed in the world each year, and so this book is offered for the consideration of all practising knee surgeons.

The challenge of unicompartmental replacement is nothing less than to replace the deformed surfaces of one compartment of the knee so effectively that the soft tissues of the whole joint, and the retained articular surfaces of the other compartments, can all resume their physiological functions. This is a more difficult task than that confronted by total knee replacement, and it is anomalous that most prosthetic designs and methods of implantation for unicompartmental replacement have remained so unsophisticated during the three decades in which the technology of total replacement has (perhaps unsteadily) advanced.

The undertaking of a unicompartmental arthroplasty requires knowledge of the mechanics of the normal knee, and of the pathological anatomy of the arthritic knee. The prosthesis used must impose no unphysiological limits on the function of the retained structures and therefore it must be implanted in a unique relationship to the ligaments of the individual knee. This may only be consistently achieved if the instruments allow measured intraoperative adjustment of the components to match the particular anatomy. The components need to be sufficiently wear resistant to function for the expected lifetime of the patient, which is usually much longer than 10 years.

Lastly, the surgeon needs to have gained the *appropriate* skills and experience. Even long familiarity with other procedures on the knee does not, it seems, suffice to avoid the consequences of the 'learning curve' for unicompartmental arthroplasty.

John Goodfellow
John O'Connor
Christopher Dodd
David Murray

Acknowledgements

Many people have assisted in the making of this book and deserve our thanks. Among them, Barbara Marks BSc (Hons) has played the central role as our organiser and has earned our admiration for her skills and our gratitude for her good humour.

We acknowledge the help and support of all our surgeon colleagues and, in particular, Peter McLardy-Smith FRCS, Roger Gundle DPhil FRCS (Orth) and Max Gibbons FRCS (Orth). Special mention has to be made of Andrew Price DPhil FRCS (Orth) who helped us to mine the wealth of information in his thesis. Hemant Pandit FRCS (Orth) gave us access to the recent clinical data he has collected and David Beard DPhil has been a constant adviser. We thank our anaesthetist colleagues, Peter Hambly FRCA, Mansukh Popat FRCA and Mathew Sainsbury FRCA for their contributions to the regime of early patient discharge. None of our clinical work would have been possible without the help of Victoria Flanagan, Cathy Jenkins, and the nurses, physiotherapists, radiographers and other staff of the Nuffield Orthopaedic Centre and we are grateful to them all.

The theoretical modelling of the human knee has been improved and refined by several "generations" of engineers and their work is frequently cited in the book. Particular mention is made of Richie Gill DPhil, Jennifer Feikes DPhil, Tung-Wu Lu DPhil and Ahmed Imran DPhil who provided invaluable help with compiling the models and animations included on the DVD.

Since 1984, the technical skills to make the implants and instruments we describe were provided by the engineers and craftsmen of Biomet UK Ltd. We specially record the many contributions of Ron Bateman during his career as Research and Development Engineering Manager in that company. David Moorse, Keith Thomas and Kit Pitman have helped in innumerable ways.

Many of the photographs were taken by Paul Cooper of the Medical Illustration Department at the Nuffield Orthopaedic Centre, and the technical diagrams are the work of Jim Stankard of Mosaic Digital Imaging Ltd.

In the past thirty years, very many professional colleagues have contributed to our studies at Oxford, as consultants, surgical trainees or engineering students, and several of their names appear as authors of papers referred to in this book.

John Goodfellow
John O'Connor
Christopher Dodd
David Murray

Contents

Introduction
Unicompartmental versus total knee replacement

Osteoarthritis of the knee is one of the most common causes of painful loss of mobility in middle-aged and elderly people in many populations and is the main indication for knee replacement surgery. From the early days of arthroplasty, it was recognized that arthritis was often limited to the medial (or lateral) compartment of the knee and, in the pioneering operation of MacIntosh [1], metal spacers could be used in one compartment or both. Gradually, however, as the advantages of bicompartmental arthroplasty were appreciated, unicompartmental replacement was less and less practised, and in some countries almost disappeared. With the introduction of tricompartmental replacement, a large body of surgical opinion concluded that osteoarthritis of the knee was a disease of the whole joint (like osteoarthritis of the hip) and that common sense required the replacement of *all* the articular surfaces to provide long-term relief of symptoms.

The attention of designers and manufacturers focused on the improvement of implants and instruments for total replacement, and the gap between the survival rates of unicompartmental knee arthroplasty (UKA) and total knee arthroplasty (TKA) widened, reinforcing the prevailing opinion of their fundamental merits.

Popular neglect of the unicompartmental alternative is reflected in a lack of innovation. The St Georg (1969) and the Marmor (1972) implants are still in use today, and most designs developed since then are very like them. Until recently, the components were implanted largely 'by eye', as in the early days of total replacement.

A further consequence of the success of TKA was loss of interest in the natural history and pathological anatomy of the osteoarthritic knee. Since total replacement is equally applicable, and almost equally successful, over the whole range of manifestations of that disease, there was no longer much point in its further analysis. However, the longitudinal studies by Ahlback [2] had already suggested that unicompartmental osteoarthritis does not inevitably spread to other parts of the knee. In addition, numerous post-mortem and intraoperative descriptions published in the 1970s and 1980s had revealed the almost universal presence of cartilage lesions in some parts of the joint in middle-aged and elderly people, implying that their presence is consistent with adequate knee function. These observations challenge the common-sense conclusion that replacement of all the articular surfaces is a necessary requirement for a clinically successful arthroplasty.

A few surgeons were able to report clinical results and cumulative survival rates to match those of total replacement, but the general opinion was (and remains) that the unicompartmental operation is more difficult than TKA and therefore less successful in the hands of the average surgeon.

If UKA is such a demanding undertaking, and if its goals of symptomatic relief and long-term survival of the implant have already been largely achieved by TKA, why change? It may, of course, offend one's sense of economy to replace more of a damaged joint than is necessary, but there are more practical reasons as well.

As to symptomatic relief, successful UKA is even more effective than successful TKA. Many surgeons who have performed both procedures have found that the range of flexion is greater and gait is more nearly normal, particularly in activities like stair climbing, because the biomechanics of the knee are more completely restored [3,4]. However, it is on the grounds of safety and reduced morbidity that unicompartmental replacement most strongly recommends itself. According to the Swedish Knee Arthroplasty Register (SKAR) 2004 report, '... the number of serious complications such as infection/arthrodesis/amputation is much less' [5]. Blood transfusion is not required and post-operative recovery is quicker [6]. Revision is usually easier after UKA than after TKA, and the results of these revisions are as good as those after primary TKA [7]. Even taking into account its lower survival rate, the shorter hospital stay of UKA makes it a more cost-effective option [7].

These advantages were documented when unicompartmental implants were usually inserted, as in total replacement, through an open approach with dislocation of the patella. It now seems that the benefits can be enhanced by the use of a minimally invasive approach, which the small size of the implant facilitates [6,8].

Unicompartmental implant design

The first 'modern' designs, the St Georg (1969) and the Marmor (1972), had polycentric metal femoral condyles articulating on flat (or nearly flat) polyethylene tibial components, both cemented to the bones [9,10] (Fig. I.1). The stated principles of Marmor's design

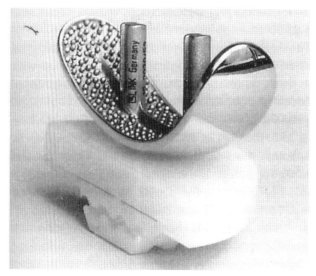

Figure I.1 St Georg unicompartmental prosthesis.

were to reproduce as accurately as possible the polycentric form of the natural femoral condyles; and to avoid constraint of the articulation by employing a non-conforming tibial plateau [11]. Most of the models introduced since were designed on the same principles.

Initially, problems were caused by wear and distortion of the thinnest polyethylene components (6 mm thick), which were abandoned in favour of thicker ones. The persisting problem of deformation of the all-polyethylene component led to the use of metal-backed tibial implants, but this, in turn, resulted in diminished thickness of polyethylene and sometimes further problems with wear [12].

In 1974, two of the authors (JWG and JJOC) introduced congruous mobile bearings for knee prostheses [13]. The first 'Oxford Knee' had a metal femoral component with a spherical articular surface, a metal tibial component which was flat, and a polyethylene mobile bearing, spherically concave above and flat below, interposed between them (Fig. I.2). The device was fully congruent at both interfaces throughout the range of movement (to minimize polyethylene wear) and fully unconstrained (to allow unrestricted movements). These features of the Oxford knee have remained unchanged to the present day.

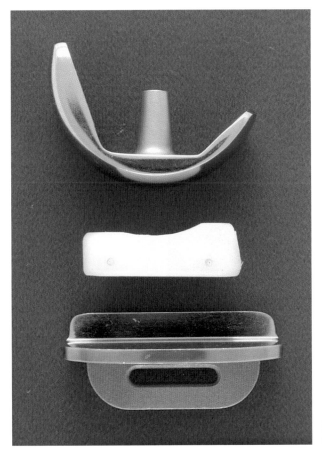

Figure I.2 The Oxford Knee (Phase 1) (1976).

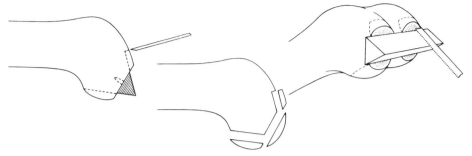

Figure I.3 Method of preparation of the femur for the Oxford Knee (Phase 1).

At first, the implant was used bicompartmentally, as a total joint replacement, but later it was used for medial or lateral unicompartmental replacement.[1] The non-articular surface of the femoral component of the original design (Phase 1) had three inclined facets and was fitted to the femur by making three saw-cuts as shown in Figure I.3.

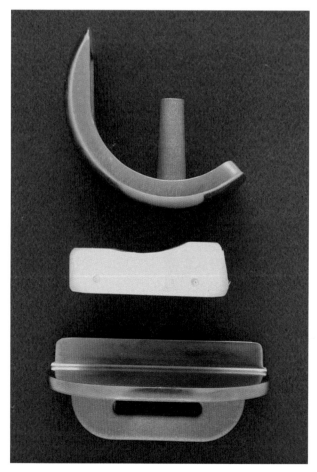

Figure I.4 The Oxford Unicompartmental Knee Arthroplasty (OUKA (Phase 2)) (1987).

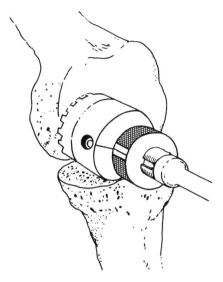

Figure I.5 Method of preparation of the femur for the OUKA (Phase 2) with a concave rotary mill turning round an adjustable spigot.

In 1987, the Phase 2 implant was introduced specifically for unicompartmental arthroplasty (OUKA)[2], medially and laterally. The non-articular surfaces of the femoral component had a flat posterior facet and a spherically concave inferior facet (Fig. I.4). The posterior femoral condyle was prepared by a saw-cut and its inferior facet was milled by a spherically concave bone-mill rotating round a spigot in a drill-hole in the condyle (Fig. I.5). By shortening the spigot, measured thicknesses of bone could be milled incrementally from the inferior surface of the condyle, allowing the ligament tensions in flexion and extension to be balanced intraoperatively and simultaneously shaping the bone to fit the implant [14].

The Phase 1 and Phase 2 prostheses were implanted through an open approach with dislocation of the patella, as in TKA. In all the long-term survival studies, Phase 1 and/or Phase 2 implants were used.

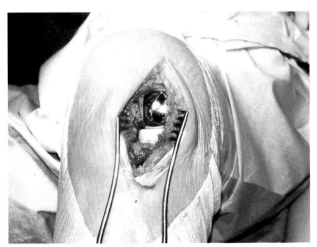

Figure I.6 The OUKA (Phase 3) (1998) implanted through a small incision.

In 1998, the Phase 3 prosthesis was introduced specifically for medial unicompartmental use with a minimally invasive approach (Fig. I.6). The single size of femoral component (used in all the Phase 1 and 2 implants) was replaced by five parametric sizes, and the universal tibial plateau was replaced by right- and left-handed tibial components. The instruments were miniaturized to facilitate their use through a small parapatellar arthrotomy, and the bearings were modified to diminish the likelihood of impingement and rotation.

Various episodes in this brief history of the implant are expanded in subsequent chapters.

Notes

1. The first unicompartmental replacement with an Oxford implant was performed by our late colleague David Fuller MS, FRCS.

2. There are precedents for our using the abbreviations TKA for total knee arthroplasty and UKA for unicompartmental knee arthroplasty, the two categories of knee replacement. By analogy, we have used OUKA for the specific procedure of Oxford unicompartmental knee arthroplasty or for the implant.

References

1. MacIntosh DL. Hemiarthroplasty of the knee using a space occupying prosthesis for painful varus and valgus deformities. *J Bone Joint Surg [Am]* 1958; **40-A**: 1431.

2. Ahlback S. Osteoarthrosis of the knee. A radiographic investigation. *Acta Radiol Diagn (Stockh)* 1968; **Suppl 277**: 7–72.

3. Laurencin CT, Zelicof SB, Scott RD, Ewald FC. Unicompartmental versus total knee arthroplasty in the same patient. A comparative study. *Clin Orthop* 1991; **273**: 151–6.

4. Rougraff BT, Heck DA, Gibson AE. A comparison of tricompartmental and unicompartmental arthroplasty for the treatment of gonarthrosis. *Clin Orthop* 1991; **273**: 157–64.

5. Lidgren L, Knutson K, Robertsson O. *Swedish Knee Arthroplasty Register: Annual Report 2004.* Lund: Swedish Knee Arthroplasty Register, 2004.

6. Price AJ, Webb J, Topf H, Dodd CA, Goodfellow JW, Murray DW. Rapid recovery after Oxford unicompartmental arthroplasty through a short incision. *J Arthroplasty* 2001; **16**: 970–6.

7. Robertsson O, Borgquist L, Knutson K, Lewold S, Lidgren L. Use of unicompartmental instead of tricompartmental prostheses for unicompartmental arthrosis in the knee is a cost-effective alternative. 15,437 primary tricompartmental prostheses were compared with 10,624 primary medial or lateral unicompartmental prostheses. *Acta Orthop Scand* 1999; **70**: 170–5.

8. Repicci JA, Eberle RW. Minimally invasive technique for unicondylar knee arthroplasty. *J South Orthop Assoc* 1999; **8**: 20–27.

9. Neider E. Schlitten prothese, Rotations knie und Scharnierprothese modell St. Georg and Endo-Modell. *Orthopäde* 1991; **20**: 170–180.

10. Marmor L. Unicompartmental and total knee arthroplasty. *Clin Orthop* 1985; **192**: 75–81.

11. Marmor L. Preface. *Prothese Unicompartimentale du Genou.* Paris: Expansion Scientifique, 1998.

12. Palmer SH, Morrison PJ, Ross AC. Early catastrophic tibial component wear after unicompartmental knee arthroplasty. *Clin Orthop* 1998; **350**: 143–8.

13. Goodfellow JW, O'Connor JJ, Shrive NG. Endoprosthetic knee joint devices. Br Patent Application 1534263, 1974.

14. Goodfellow JW, O'Connor JJ. Oxford Knee (femoral). UK, French, German, Swiss Patent EP 0327397, Irish Patent 62951, US Patent 5314482, 1989.

Design of the Oxford Knee

The description of the Oxford Knee starts with an explanation of the function of mobile bearings in knee prostheses. An obvious advantage is that the areas of contact between the joint surfaces are maximized, and wear at the polyethylene surfaces is diminished.

Part 1 Designing against wear

Articular surface shapes and contact pressures

Most surface replacements of the knee, total as well as unicompartmental, have articular surfaces like those shown in Figure 1.1, approximating to the shapes of the ends of the human femur and tibia. The metal femoral surfaces are convex and the polyethylene tibial surfaces are flat or shallowly concave. These shapes do not fit one another, in any relative position, and so only parts of their articular surfaces are in contact and able to transmit load.

Most prosthetic femoral condyles attempt to mimic nature and are polyradial, with the shortest radius posterior. Thus the area of contact is smaller in flexion than in extension (Fig. 1.1). However, the compressive loads transmitted across the interface are potentially greatest in flexion, attaining up to six times body weight during stair ascent and descent [1].

For a given load, the average contact pressure (load per unit area) at the articular surfaces is inversely proportional to the area of contact; therefore the less congruous the surfaces, the higher is the average pressure at their interface. The wear rate of ultra-high-molecular-weight polyethylene (referred to hereafter as 'polyethylene') increases exponentially with increasing contact pressure, rather than linearly as would be expected from classical wear theory [2]; conversely, wear rate decreases with increasing contact area [3].

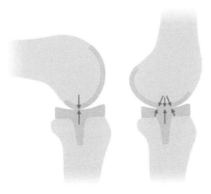

Figure 1.1 Typical polycentric incongruous knee replacement.

The natural knee

The presence of the cartilaginous menisci in the knee of humans (and of all other mammals) gives rise to an entirely different regime of contact (Fig. 1.2). Instead of one incongruous interface, two congruous interfaces are created, with much better distribution of load.

Fairbank, in 1948, first deduced that the human meniscus had a load-bearing function [4] and suggested the mechanism of load transmission shown in Figure 1.3. The menisci consist mainly of collagen fibres disposed circumferentially to withstand the tensile hoop stresses engendered by load bearing; these stresses are resisted at the anterior and posterior horns by their attachments to the tibia [5]. The proportion of load transmitted indirectly by the menisci in human (and animal) joints has been estimated as between 45 and 70 per cent of the applied load [6]. The remaining 30–55 per cent is carried by the articular cartilage of the femoral and tibial surfaces through their direct contact in the middle third of each plateau.

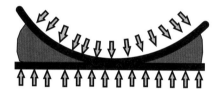

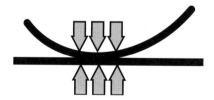

Figure 1.2 Load-sharing function of the meniscus, increasing effective contact area and reducing contact pressure. Loss of a meniscus reduces contact area and increases contact pressure.

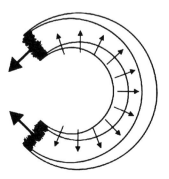

Figure 1.3 Mechanism of load transmission: the radially outward component of applied pressure is resisted by hoop stresses in the circumferential fibres of the meniscus. (Adapted from and reproduced with permission from Lippincott Williams & Wilkins [Shrive NG, O'Connor JJ and Goodfellow JW. Load-bearing in the knee joint. *Clin Orthop* 1978; **131**: 279–87].)

Mobility of the natural meniscus

Anteroposterior movements of the femoral condyles on the tibia during flexion–extension and axial rotation have to be accommodated by movements of the menisci. In 1680 Borelli [7] noticed that 'they are pulled forward when the knee is extended and backwards in flexion'. Various estimates and measurements of these movements during flexion have been reported: 6 mm medially and 12 mm laterally [8]; 5.1 mm (SD 0.96) medially and 11.2 mm (SD 2.29) laterally [9]; medial anterior horn 7.1 mm (SD 2.49), medial posterior horn 3.9 mm (SD 1.75), lateral anterior horn 9.5 mm (SD 3.96), and lateral posterior horn 5.6 mm (SD 2.76) [10].

Compliance of the natural meniscus

During flexion–extension and axial rotation, the natural meniscus not only changes its position on the tibial plateau, as the movements of the femoral condyle dictate, but also changes shape to fit the various curvatures of the polyradial femoral condyle (Fig. 1.4). In full extension, the large radius of the inferior surface of the condyle forces the limbs of the meniscus apart in an anteroposterior direction. As the knee flexes, and the smaller radius of the posterior condyle is offered, the anteroposterior measurement of the meniscus diminishes appropriately, possibly because divergence of the tibiofemoral contact areas forces the two menisci apart, drawing their anterior and posterior limbs closer together (Fig. 1.5) [6]. Changes in the shapes of the menisci are reflected in the differences in anteroposterior movements of the anterior and posterior horns and in the mediolateral movements of the medial and lateral edges of the two menisci observed by Vedi *et al.* [10].

Discussion

The meniscus is an integral part of the tibial articular surface, serving to maximize the contact area without limiting angular and translational movement between the bones. Therefore load is transmitted at an average pressure that the articular cartilage can withstand. Evidence of the importance of this mechanism is provided by the observation that excision (or dysfunction) of a meniscus results in osteoarthritic degeneration of the remaining cartilage surfaces in the affected compartment [4].

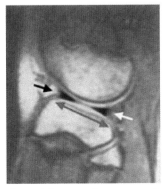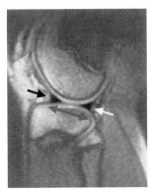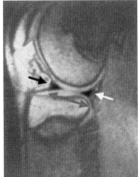

Figure 1.4 Magnetic resonance images demonstrating changes in the anteroposterior span of the meniscus during flexion. (Adapted from and reproduced with permission and copyright © of the British Editorial Society of Bone and Joint Surgery [Vedi V, Williams A, Tennant SJ, Spouse E, Hunt DM, Gedroyc WM. Meniscal movement. An in vivo study using dynamic MRI. *J. Bone Joint Surg [Br]* 1999; **81-B**: 37–41].)

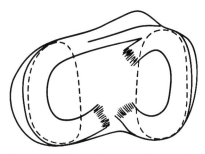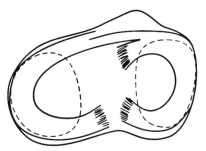

Figure 1.5 Shape changes of the meniscus during flexion-extension. Dotted curves outline contact areas in extension (left) and flexion (right) (diagramatic). (Reproduced with permission from Lippincott Williams & Wilkins [from Shrive N G, O'Connor JJ, and Goodfellow JW. Load-bearing in the knee joint. *Clin Orthop* 1978; **131**: 279–87].)

The Oxford "Meniscal" Knee

The mechanical advantages conferred by the natural meniscus can be enjoyed by an artificial knee if it is provided with two joint interfaces instead of one. The design of the articular surfaces of the Oxford Knee has not changed since its first implantation in 1976 (Fig. 1.6). The meniscofemoral interface (ball-in-socket) allows the angular movements of flexion–extension, the meniscotibial interface (flat-on-flat) allows translational movements (Fig. 1.7), and axial rotation is allowed by a combination of translation and spinning movement at both interfaces. The unconstrained mobile bearing does not resist the movements demanded by the soft tissues, muscles, and ligaments, and its surfaces experience mainly compressive forces normal to these surfaces, features which should minimize component loosening [11].

The method of load transmission through the polyethylene bearing is, of course, quite different from that through the natural meniscus, but the functions of the two structures are analogous. The prosthetic bearing converts one incongruous interface into two congruous interfaces, maximizing the area available for load transmission without limiting the freedom of joint movement, a feature which should minimize polyethylene

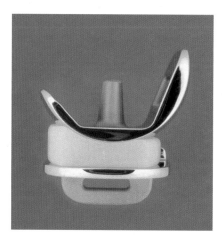

Figure 1.6 Components of the Oxford Knee (Phase 1).

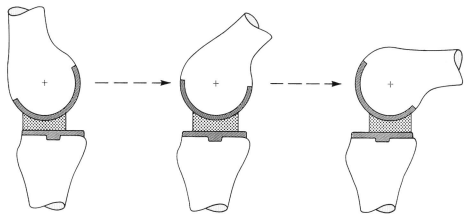

Figure 1.7 Combined sliding at the femoro-meniscal and menisco-tibial interfaces during flexion–extension, maintaining full conformity between the components in all positions. (Reproduced from Goodfellow JW, O'Connor JJ, Murray DW "Principles of meniscal bearing arthroplasty for unicompartmental knee replacement" In: Ph Cartier, JA Epinette, G Deschamps & Ph Hernigou Eds. *Cahiers d'enseignement de la SOFCOT* 61 "Unicompartmental Knee Arthroplasty", 1997: 174–180 (permission requested).)

wear while restoring physiological function. These are the justifications for calling the Oxford Knee a 'meniscal bearing' implant.

Why use a spherical not a polyradial femoral condyle?

A rigid polyethylene bearing can model only the mobility of the natural meniscus, and not its compliance. It cannot change shape and therefore cannot fit more than one of the several radii offered by a polyradial condyle. The only pairs of shapes that can maintain congruity in all relative positions of the components are a sphere in a spherical socket and a flat surface on a flat surface. Figure 1.8 shows the medial half of a specimen of a distal femur, sectioned through the sulcus of the trochlear groove. A circle fits the cartilage surface at the base of the trochlear groove quite well. Another circle fits the posterior facets of the femoral condyle, although it does not match its most distal facet. Therefore a spherical femoral prosthesis can reproduce the shape of all but the most anterior part of the medial condyle.

Other mobile-bearing designs

Since 1978, several designers have used mobile bearings in total and unicompartmental knee prostheses but with polyradial femoral condyles [12]. In such implants, the concavity on the upper surface of the bearing must have a radius of curvature large enough to accommodate the largest radius of the femoral condyle (offered in extension) and therefore too large to match the smaller radii (offered in all positions of flexion when the compression forces between the components are greater). Thus the function of such a mobile bearing is not analogous to that of the natural meniscus and is unlikely to minimize wear. Non-conforming mobile-bearing prostheses offer little theoretical advantage over non-conforming fixed-bearing designs.

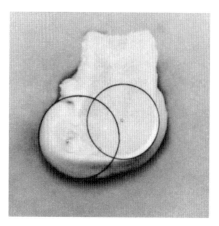

Figure 1.8 Sagittal section of the distal femur demonstrating that the sulcus of the trochlea and most of the medial condyle are circular. (This material has been reproduced from the *Journal of Engineering in Medicine: Proceedings of the Institution of Mechanical Engineers* Part H. 1989 Vol 216 Issue H4 pp 223–233. The geometry of the knee in the sagittal plane. O'Connor J, Goodfellow J, Shercliff T, Biden E. Permission is granted by the Council of the Institution of Mechanical Engineers.)

Polyethylene wear in the Oxford Knee

The following studies have demonstrated that the theoretical expectation of a low polyethylene wear rate has been fulfilled in practice.

Retrieval studies

Twenty-three bearings were retrieved from 18 failed bicompartmental Oxford arthroplasties, 1–9 years after implantation [13]. The minimum thickness of each was measured with a dial gauge (Fig. 1.9) and compared with the mean thickness of 25 unused bearings. The mean penetration rate was very low; calculated by two methods, it was either 0.043 or 0.026 mm/year. There was no correlation between the initial thickness of the bearings (range 3.5–10.5 mm) and their rate of wear.

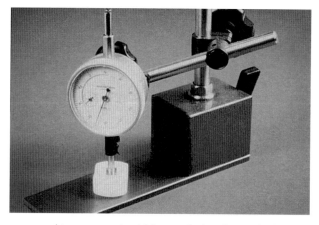

Figure 1.9 Dial gauge used to measure the thickness of a bearing at the bottom of the spherical socket. (Reproduced with permission and copyright © of the British Editorial Society of Bone and Joint Surgery [Psychoyios V, Crawford RW, O'Connor JJ, Murray DW. Wear of congruent meniscal bearings in unicompartmental knee arthroplasty. A retrieval study of 16 specimens. *J Bone Joint Surg [Br]* 1998; **80-B**: 876–82].)

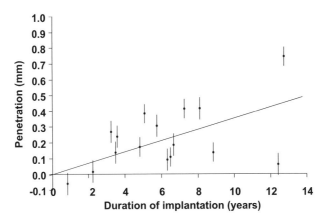

Figure 1.10 Retrieval studies. Measured penetration into the bearing plotted against duration of implantation. The vertical line through each data point represents one standard deviation of the mean of the measured thickness of unused bearings obtained direct from the manufacturer. The regression line through the data gives the penetration rate (mm/year). (Reproduced with permission and copyright © of the British Editorial Society of Bone and Joint Surgery [Psychoyios V, Crawford RW, O'Connor JJ, Murray DW. Wear of congruent meniscal bearings in unicompartmental knee arthroplasty. A retrieval study of 16 specimens. *J Bone Joint Surg [Br]* 1998; **80-B**: 876–82].)

The same method was used to study 16 bearings retrieved from failed OUKA (Phase 2) medial arthroplasties, 0.8–12.8 years after implantation [14]. The mean penetration rate was 0.036 mm/year (maximum 0.08) (Fig. 1.10). Again, there was no correlation between the rate of wear and the initial bearing thickness (range 3.5–11.5 mm).

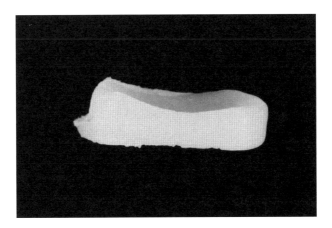

Figure 1.11 Retrieved bearing showing damage due to anterior impingement. (Reproduced with permission and copyright © of the British Editorial Society of Bone and Joint Surgery [Psychoyios V, Crawford RW, O'Connor JJ, Murray DW. Wear of congruent meniscal bearings in unicompartmental knee arthroplasty. A retrieval study of 16 specimens. *J Bone Joint Surg [Br]* 1998; **80-B**: 876–82].)

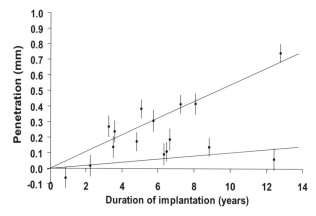

Figure 1.12 Retrieval studies. Penetration against duration of implantation for bearings with (upper line) and without (lower line) evidence of impingement. (Reproduced with permission and copyright © of the British Editorial Society of Bone and Joint Surgery [Psychoyios V, Crawford RW, O'Connor JJ, Murray DW. Wear of congruent meniscal bearings in unicompartmental knee arthroplasty. A retrieval study of 16 specimens. *J Bone Joint Surg [Br]* 1998; **80-B**: 876–82].)

Ten bearings had erosion of their non-articular surfaces, caused by impingement against bone or cement. The most common site was anterior, produced by impingement in extension against bone in front of the femoral component (Fig. 1.11). The six bearings without impingement had a mean penetration rate of 0.01 mm/year compared with 0.054 mm/year for the 10 bearings with impingement ($P < 0.0001$) (Fig. 1.12).

Price [15] used the same method to study a further 47 Phase 1 and Phase 2 bearings retrieved after OUKA at a mean time to revision of 8.4 years (SD 4.1). Twenty had been implanted for more than 10 years (maximum 17 years). Thirty-one of the 47 bearings showed evidence of impingement, and the mean penetration rate in these was 0.07 mm/year. The rate for the 16 bearings without impingement was 0.01 mm/year, the same as that found by Psychoyios *et al.* [14]. The penetration rate of Phase 1 bearings (machined from blocks of Hostulen RCH1000 polyethylene) was about double that of Phase 2 bearings (individually compression moulded from Montel Hifax 1900H powder). However, the impingement rate in Phase 1 implants (98 per cent) was also much higher than in Phase 2 implants (58 per cent).

In vivo penetration studies using Röntgen stereometric analysis

We have developed a method of measuring wear *in vivo* using Röntgen stereometric analysis, and have applied it to patients following OUKA [15,16]. The method does not require markers attached to the components or implanted in the patient's bones and therefore can be used retrospectively. Penetration of the bearings was measured in eight controls (3 weeks after OUKA) and in seven patients in whom the prosthesis had been implanted about 10 years previously [17] (Fig. 1.13). The mean penetration for the control group was 0.1 mm, demonstrating the accuracy of the

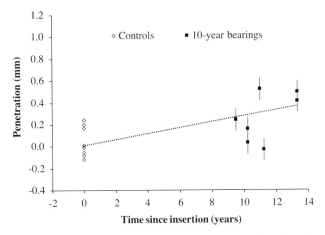

Figure 1.13 RSA studies. Penetration into bearings plotted against time since insertion for a group of patients with minimum 9.5 year follow-up and a group of controls measured immediately postoperatively. (Reproduced with permission and copyright © of the British Editorial Society of Bone and Joint Surgery [Price A J, Short A, Kellet C, et al. Ten year *in vivo* wear measurement of a fully congruent mobile bearing unicompartmental knee arthroplasty. *J Bone Joint Surg [Br]* 2005; **87-B**: 1493–97].)

method (Fig. 1.13). The mean penetration rate for the 10-year group was 0.02 mm/year, similar to that observed in retrieved bearings without impingement (0.01 mm/year).

Wear simulation studies

Retrieval and *in vivo* studies are the 'gold standard', providing evidence of actual performance of components in the infinitely varied circumstances of real life. Simulation studies have the disadvantage that the tests may be so far from lifelike as to invalidate the results. However, they are useful for longitudinal measurement of wear, for comparison of competing designs and materials under similarly controlled conditions, and for simulating the effects of years of natural wear in a few months.

A Stanmore knee simulator [18] was used to test a group of OUKA bearings over 4 million cycles [19]. During the first million cycles (thought to represent 1 year of normal activity), the bearings had a measured penetration of 0.05 mm (Fig. 1.14). Thereafter the penetration rate was steady at 0.019 mm/year. The early higher rate of penetration was attributed to creep of the viscoelastic polyethylene which ceased once the bearings had bedded in after about a million cycles.

Finite-element analysis

Morra and Greenwald [20] carried out a finite-element stress analysis of four unicompartmental prostheses, two fixed-bearing and two mobile-bearing (the OUKA and an implant with a polycentric femoral component). They modelled three instants in the normal walking cycle with the knee near extension, and calculated surface contact areas and pressures and the maximum value of the von Mises stress, said to be a measure of the tendency for delamination.

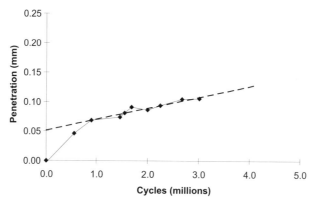

Figure 1.14 Simulator studies. Measured penetration plotted against millions of cycles of movement and load, with a regression line through the >1 million cycle data. (Reproduced, with permission, from Scott R, Schroeder D. Correlation of knee simulation to in-vivo use: evaluating the Oxford Unicompartmental knee. *Transactions of the Orthopaedic Research Society* **vol. 25**, Orlando, Florida, 2000; 434.)

As expected, the fixed-bearing designs both had small contact areas, high contact stresses, and von Mises stresses significantly in excess of the material damage threshold (9 MPa). Both mobile-bearing knees had contact areas at least three times larger than the fixed-bearing designs but smaller than their nominal values because of manufacturing tolerances. The contact areas of the OUKA implant varied from 284 to 346 mm², compared with the nominal value of 580 mm² for ideally shaped components. Both mobile-bearing designs exhibited '... very low contact stress and an absence of von Mises stress above the material damage threshold'. No calculations were performed for knees flexed to 90°–100°, when the loads can be larger and the contact areas of the polycentric mobile bearing prosthesis would have been smaller than those of the congruent OUKA.

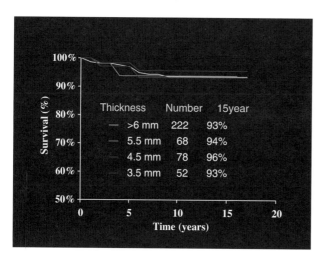

Figure 1.15 Survival curves for patients with different thicknesses of bearing; cumulative survival rate plotted against postoperative years. (Unpublished data reproduced with the permission of Mr A J Price.)

Survival analysis

The survival curves of 420 OUKAs (Phases 1, 2, and 3) stratified according to bearing thickness [15] showed that the long-term survival rate was independent of the thickness of polyethylene (Fig. 1.15).

Discussion

The gradual diminution of bearing thickness over time is due to a combination of **creep** (bulk cold-flow of the viscoelastic polymer) and loss of material due to **wear** at its two articular surfaces. Penetration measurements of retrieved bearings do not allow an estimate of the relative contributions of these two processes, but the simulator studies suggest that creep only occurs initially and that, thereafter, penetration can be attributed entirely to surface wear.

Penetration rate

There was a significantly higher penetration rate in bearings with evidence of impingement, possibly because bone and polyethylene debris in the joint acted as third bodies between the articular surfaces. Impingement can be avoided by appropriate surgical technique, and a properly implanted bearing should not impinge against bone or cement.

The mean rate of penetration of the 22 medial bearings with no evidence of impingement, the rate measured *in vivo* at 10 years in clinically successful patients, and the rate in the simulator studies were all very small (0.01–0.02 mm/year). They are an order of magnitude lower than the mean rate of 0.15 mm/year reported for the St Georg, the only fixed-bearing implant for which there are comparable retrieval data [21]. It is not wise to extrapolate long-term wear rates from short-term measurements because the polymer may degrade, but, at the rates reported, the OUKA bearings would lose 1 mm of thickness in 50–100 years. The high survival rates of the OUKA up to 17 years after implantation demonstrate that, in congruous articulation, polyethylene can survive as long as the patient even when used in thin components (see Fig. 1.15).

The rate of penetration of the Oxford bearings was also much lower than that reported by Wroblewski [22] for the acetabular component of the fully congruous Charnley hip (0.19 mm/year). This is not surprising as the projected area of contact is larger in the OUKA than in the Charnley hip, and the contact stresses are correspondingly lower.

A similarly low rate of penetration (0.026 mm/year) was found for a fixed-bearing total knee prosthesis with fully congruent cylindrical articular surfaces [23], suggesting that it is congruity, rather than the use of mobile bearings, that allows the transmission of high loads with little wear.

Similar data have not been published for mobile bearings articulating with polyradial femoral condyles, but they may not enjoy such low wear rates as they cannot be congruent throughout the range of movement. In one such device, the most frequent cause for revision was bearing failure, and bearing exchange for wear is a well-recognized procedure [24,25].

Bearing thickness

In incongruent articulations, the wear rate of polyethylene is greater when it is used in a thin layer [26]. Perhaps the most important observation made during our retrieval studies, with particular significance for unicompartmental arthroplasty, is that polyethylene used in congruent articulation has a wear rate (and a survival rate) that is independent of its initial thickness, at least down to 3.5 mm (see Fig. 1.15). This fact is less important in TKA where more extensive bone removal allows the use of thick tibial implants, but it is of consequence in unicompartmental prostheses when preservation of bone stock and minimal invasion are required. In fixed-bearing UKA designs, it is thought unsafe to use a polyethylene layer thinner than 6 mm [27]. However, a congruous meniscal bearing that is only 3.5 mm thick at its thinnest point wears no more rapidly than a thicker one.

Volumetric wear

Penetration (linear wear plus creep) is not the only measure of wear. Another measure is the volume of debris generated (volumetric wear). Volumetric wear increases in proportion to the area of contact but, since it reduces with reduction in penetration, the beneficial effect of the low contact pressure at congruous surfaces may more than balance the adverse effect of their large contact areas. Calculations of the mean volume of wear debris produced at the articular surfaces of the Oxford bearing give a figure of about 6 mm^3/year (for bearings without impingement). The St Georg fixed-bearing implant had a measured volumetric wear rate of 17.3 mm^3/year [21]. No comparable data are available for other knee replacements, but the volumetric acetabular wear rates (assessed *in vivo*) for various designs of hip prosthesis, which also have congruous surfaces, vary from 26 to 89 mm^3/year [28]. The tissues around the hip are believed to be able to tolerate a mean of 600 mm^3 of polyethylene debris before bone resorption necessitates revision [29].

Therefore it is unlikely that the volume of wear particles from a properly functioning meniscal bearing will cause problems. However, with the accelerated wear rate associated with impingement, it is possible that particle debris accumulated in the long term might become great enough to cause osteolysis.

There is a suspicion that it is the very small particles generated by wear at congruous surfaces that cause osteolysis and aseptic loosening. However, Price's study [15] of 47 retrieved Oxford bearings showed that even those most damaged by impingement came from knees with no evidence of osteolysis. Sathasivam *et al.* [3] stated that 'there is no disadvantage with regard to particle size or type associated with large contact areas'. The survival rates better than 90 per cent at 17 years (see Fig. 1.15) also imply an absence of significant osteolysis.

The debris generated by extra-articular impingement probably consists of larger particles. These may act as third bodies and hasten wear, as suggested by the observed correlation of impingement and increased penetration. The surgeon needs to take all necessary precautions to avoid impingement.

Part 2 Restoring natural mobility and stability

The shapes of the articular surfaces of the Oxford Knee components do not match those of either compartment of the natural joint and, even if they did, they could hardly be expected to match exactly the shapes of the surfaces of each individual patient. How is it possible for such an implant to restore normal mobility and stability, normal mechanics and kinematics?

The complex three-dimensional pattern of movement of the natural knee depends upon the following:

(1) the shapes of its articular surfaces;

(2) the design of the array of ligaments that hold the bones together;

(3) the magnitude and direction of the forces applied by muscle contraction in response to gravity and ground reaction.

In any particular joint, features (1) and (2) are constant and therefore the movements of the **unloaded** knee should be predictable and repeatable. However, the forces applied during activity are as infinitely variable as the uses to which the human limb is put, and the consequent patterns of movement of the **loaded** knee are also infinitely varied.

The unloaded human knee

The pattern of movement of the unloaded knee is highly ordered. In a study in which the movements were controlled solely by the intact ligaments and articular surfaces, 12 unloaded cadaver specimens were passively flexed and extended [30]. The femur rotated 22° (SD 7°) externally during flexion, and internally by the same amount during extension. In every test, the bones followed a single unique path on each other, with a direct relationship between flexion angle and obligatory axial rotation (the 'screw-home mechanism') (Fig. 1.16). This pattern was readily disturbed by any applied load or torque, but the bones returned to their preferred path when the load was removed.

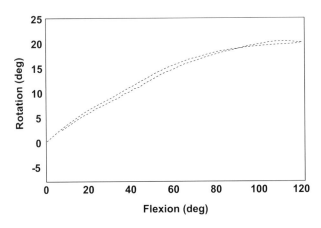

Figure 1.16 External rotation of the femur plotted against flexion angle demonstrating that the path followed during flexion was accurately retraced during extension. (Reproduced from the DPhil Thesis of JD Feikes [35].)

Ligaments

The role of the ligaments in controlling this pattern of movement is readily demonstrated. Ligament sectioning studies [31–34] have established that the anterior cruciate ligament (ACL) is the primary constraint upon anterior tibial translation (and a secondary constraint on internal tibial rotation) and the posterior cruciate ligament (PCL) is the primary constraint on posterior tibial translation (and a secondary constraint on external tibial rotation). The collateral ligaments are the primary constraints on abduction and adduction and on internal rotation (medial collateral ligament (MCL)) and external rotation (lateral collateral ligament (LCL)).

Articular surfaces

During the cadaver studies referred to above, three further specimens showed disorderly movements (Fig. 1.17). On subsequent dissection, two were found to have articular surfaces eroded by disease (Figs. 1.17(a) and 1.17(b)) and one had partial division of the MCL (Fig. 1.17(c)). For each specimen, the path followed during flexion was very different from that followed in extension, and the angle of axial rotation was no longer uniquely coupled to the flexion angle. These specimens, which no longer had any preferred path, did not resist being positioned anywhere between the upper and lower curves.

The role of the articular surfaces is more difficult to study than that of the ligaments because it is not possible to alter the shape of an articular facet without simultaneously making some ligament fibres slack (causing instability) or tightening others (causing limitation of movement). Therefore, unlike the ligaments, no particular movement constraint can be attributed to any particular feature of joint surface shape, *the function of the articular surfaces being mainly to keep the ligaments at their appropriate tension by resisting interpenetration.* As we shall see, prosthetic articular surfaces, if they reproduce *only* this function, can restore normal movement even if they are not shaped exactly like the natural surfaces.

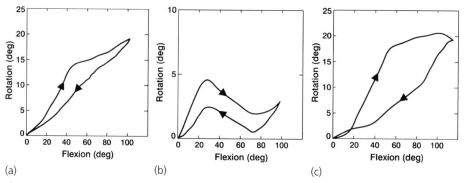

(a) (b) (c)

Figure 1.17 External femoral rotation plotted against flexion angle for three specimens: (a) and (b) had severe osteoarthritic lesions, and (c) had a partially divided MCL. (Reproduced from the DPhil Thesis of JD Feikes [35].)

Movement of the contact points

It is obvious that, during flexion, the points of contact on the femur move from the inferior surfaces of the femoral condyles to their posterior surfaces. However, the positions of the contact points on the tibial plateau are less obvious because of the presence of the menisci. Radiographic studies are not ideal because cartilage is radiolucent, and MRI is unreliable as the fine detail of the contacting surfaces can be trapped within one line of pixels on the VDU monitor. Load deforms the cartilage surfaces and the menisci, and creates areas, not points, of contact. These technical problems may account for some of the variability in descriptions of the contact regime.

The point of closest approach of the round surface of the femoral condyle to the flatter tibial plateau can be taken as the 'contact point' in each compartment. Feikes [35] digitized points on the articular surfaces in relation to the bone shafts in cadavers and then used bone movement data, like that in Figure 1.16, for computer reconstruction of the positions of the contact points. She found that during 120° of flexion the contact points moved backwards 7.8 mm (SD 7.4) medially and 12.1 mm (SD 2.2) laterally. The movements occurred continuously over the range of flexion. Walker et al. [36] had used a similar method to study contact point movement in the loaded knee (see page 23).

Movement of the condyle centres

Iwaki et al. [37] analysed sagittal plane MRI images of (nominally) unloaded cadaver knees. The centre of a circle fitted to the image of the lateral condyle moved backwards by 19 mm on a straight line fitted to the (convex) lateral plateau. Two intersecting circles were fitted to the image of the (polyradial) medial condyle, and two intersecting straight lines to the (concave) medial plateau. The centre of the anterior medial circle remained stationary on the anterior facet of the tibia during flexion from −5° to +5°; the centre of the posterior medial circle then moved backwards about 3 mm during flexion from 5° to 120°.

However, Iwaki et al. showed a discontinuity of 8 mm in the positions of the medial condyle centres as contact moved from the anterior facet to the posterior facet fitted to the tibial plateau. They interpreted this as evidence that the posterior movement of the condyle was due to its rocking, not rolling, on the tibia. However, the apparent discontinuity could have arisen from their use of two circles and two straight lines to represent the articular surfaces, with the slopes of each pair changing discontinuously at their points of intersection. Rehder [38] measured sagittal sections of the medial and lateral femoral condyles and fitted continuous curves to each with an accuracy of ± 0.2 mm. He observed no discontinuities in shape.

If the supposed discontinuity is ignored, the sum of the backward movement of the medial condyle during 125° flexion, whether as the result of rocking or rolling, is more than 8 mm.

These movements of the centres of the condyles are not the same as the movements of the contact points. The medial tibial plateau is concave and the lateral tibial plateau is convex, each of radius about 70 mm [8]. The two femoral condyles have radii of about 20 mm. From the geometry of a small circle moving in contact with a large concave or convex circle, it is easy to show that the medial condyle centre moves about 30 per cent less than its contact point and the lateral centre about 30 per cent more than its contact point. Measuring from Figure 6 of the paper by Iwaki *et al.* [37], the diagram records a mean movement of 7.1 mm posteriorly of the medial condyle centre (including the discontinuity) and 23.5 mm posteriorly of the lateral condyle centre. By our calculations, this is equivalent to contact point movements of 9.2 mm medially and 16.5 mm laterally. These distances compare with contact point movements of 7.8 mm (SD 7.4) medially and 12.1 mm (SD 2.2) laterally reported by Feikes [35]. Iwaki *et al.* [37] do not report standard deviations but the calculated mean values of their contact point movements are reasonably consistent with those of Feikes. It seems that the data provided by Iwaki *et al.*, although interpreted differently by those authors, is consistent with the concept of rollback, medially as well as laterally.

Discussion

In unloaded knees, as far as possible free from the effects of intrinsic and extrinsic loads, passive movements are controlled solely by the shapes of the articular surfaces and the design of the ligaments. The pattern of these movements is constant and repeatable. Flexion and extension are coupled to obligatory rotation and require backward translation of the contact areas on the tibia in flexion ('rollback'), with the medial contact area moving less than the lateral contact area.

Thus in these artificial unloaded circumstances there is a 'normal pattern of movement' of the human knee which a prosthesis can either restore or not.

The unloaded prosthetic knee

It is only in the laboratory, using a rig with six degrees of freedom and the weight of the bones counterbalanced, that it is possible to be sure of moving the knee without applying load to stretch its ligaments or indent its articular surfaces. However, passive movements performed by the clinician while supporting the limb, particularly in anaesthetized subjects without muscle tone, can be similar to the unloaded state of the laboratory preparation.

In 1978, we reported that in cadaver specimens with Oxford implants, forward movement of the bearing (from the rolled back position) was essential to the movement of extension and that, if bearing movement was blocked, extension was also blocked [11]. It was recently shown in the operating room, by tensometer measurements during medial OUKA, that a force of 150 N applied to the front of a medial bearing was not sufficient to prevent it moving forward during passive extension of the leg (Shakespeare 2006, to be published).

Bearing movements have also been measured using fluoroscopy in patients with medial OUKA after wound closure while they were still anaesthetized (Price, personal communication). In the patient whose movements are recorded in Figure 1.19 below, the bearing moved backwards 9 mm during passive flexion to 125° both under anaesthesia and when awake 6 months postoperatively.

Bradley *et al.* [39] compared lateral radiographs of the knee in extension and in 90° flexion up to 5 years after OUKA (medial or lateral). The films were taken with the subjects lying on their side on the X-ray table with the muscles relaxed. The mean position of the bearings in flexion was 4.4 mm (range 0–13.5) posterior to their position in extension medially and 6.0 mm (range 1.6–13.0) laterally.

Discussion

In the anaesthetized patient, the only forces available to thrust the medial bearing forwards with the power that Shakespeare measured are the compressive forces at the articular surfaces and the tensile forces in the ligaments, both engendered by the force that the examiner applied in attempting to extend the leg.

The movements of the bearings in the prosthetic joint, immediately after implantation and without muscle tone, were similar to the movements of the contact areas in the unloaded natural knee.

The radiographic study at a longer follow-up time showed that bearings continue to move in the same sense for at least 5 years after implantation. The mean movement was about half that seen intraoperatively and the spread of the data was greater.

The loaded human knee

The unloaded knee behaves in a predictable fashion because its articular surfaces do not alter their shapes and the ligaments do not alter their lengths. When significant loads are applied, both these things happen. Ligaments stretch under tension and articular surfaces indent under compression, changing the constraints to movement and profoundly modifying, even reversing, the underlying pattern described above.

Walker et al. [36] studied the movements of the contact points in cadaver knees in an apparatus similar to that used by Feikes [35] but with the specimen loaded by a weight hung from an intramedullary rod in the femoral shaft and resisted by tension in a wire sewn to the quadriceps tendon. Using the same methods of analysis of the measurements as Feikes, they found that during the first 45° of flexion the contact points moved backwards on the tibia by 13 mm (SD 3) medially and 14 mm (SD 3) laterally, with no movement on further flexion. The patterns of movement differed in the two experiments which themselves differed only by the presence or absence of load and tissue deformation. Kurosawa and Walker [40] used the same apparatus to study femoral condyle movements. During flexion to 75°, the mean movement of the centres of the medial femoral condyles was forwards 4.5 mm (SD 2.1), and then backwards 2.3 mm (SD 2.8) during flexion to 120°. The centres of the lateral condyles moved steadily backwards by a mean of 17.0 mm (SD 5.5) during flexion. The differential movements of the medial and lateral centres implied external rotation of the femur of 20.2° (SD 6).

The loaded prosthetic knee

Patellar tendon angle

The patellar tendon angle (PTA) is the angle in the sagittal plane between the tendon and the long axis of the tibia. Because of its central location in the knee, it is little affected by axial rotation and gives an indirect measure of sagittal plane kinematics. The tendon rotates posteriorly during flexion, moving steadily backwards about its insertion into the tibial tubercle.

It was shown in cadaver studies [41] that the normal pattern of PTA was restored throughout the range of flexion after medial OUKA with both cruciates preserved. After

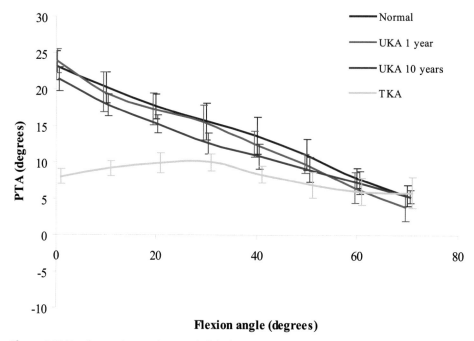

Figure 1.18 Patellar tendon angle recorded during a step-up exercise and plotted against flexion angle for groups of 5 normal volunteers, 5 patients one year and 5 patients 10 years after medial OUKA, and 5 patients one year after PCL-retaining TKA. [15]. (Reproduced from the DPhil Thesis of AJ Price).

TKA with an unconstrained fixed-bearing prosthesis (implanted after division of the ACL), anterior subluxation of the femur caused an increase in the PTA in high flexion, i.e. loss of the normal rollback. When a posterior stabilized TKA was implanted after division of both cruciates, the PTA became normal in flexion as the cam of the prosthesis artificially restored natural rollback.

Price *et al.* [42] used dynamic fluoroscopy to measure the PTA in the knees of five patients at 1 year after OUKA and five patients at 10 years. The measurements were compared with the knees of five patients who had undergone TKA and five normal volunteers (Fig. 1.18). The graphs show no significant difference in the pattern of tendon movement between the control knees and those with OUKA. In contrast, the sagittal plane mechanics after TKA were significantly disturbed.

Bearing movement *in vivo*

Price *et al.* (unpublished data) also measured bearing movement fluoroscopically during active extension/flexion and during step-up (Fig. 1.19). Movements in activity were very different from those measured passively. The backward movements of the bearing during *passive* flexion at 6 months were quite similar to those measured under anaesthesia 6 months earlier, but the bearing moved forwards on the tibia during *active* flexion to 25° and then remained more or less stationary during further flexion to 100°. However, during step-up the bearing moved forwards during flexion to 75° and then backwards during subsequent flexion. Bearing movement, therefore, is activity dependent.

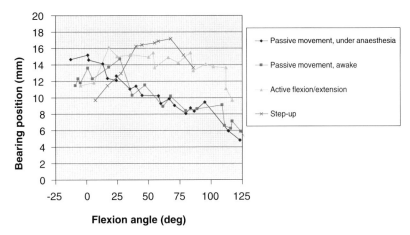

Figure 1.19 Bearing position during passive and active movements plotted against flexion angle for a single patient. (Unpublished data, reproduced with permission of AJ Price and JV Baré.)

Gait analysis

Jefferson and Whittle [43] assessed a group of medial OUKA patients in the gait labora-tory. Seven parameters of their normal level walking gait (speed, cadence, stride length, sagittal plane and coronal plane angles, and sagittal plane and abduction moments) were compared with those of a group of age- and sex-matched volunteers with no locomotor problems. All seven parameters of the patients' gait were restored to the normal range.

Discussion

Since there is no single pattern of knee movement under load, it is difficult to ensure that comparisons before and after surgery are valid. The pattern of forces can only be adequately regulated to produce repeatable patterns of movement with very simple defined activities, such as straight leg raise, step-up, etc.

The evidence of cadaver studies is that the anatomical features of the joint (the shapes of its articular surfaces and the design of its ligaments) define the envelope within which the bones are moved by the very large extrinsic and intrinsic forces. These forces can either reinforce or reverse the pattern of contact in the unloaded joint, implying that the detailed shapes of the articular surfaces allow rather than control the site of their contact areas. If the main function of the natural surface shapes is to maintain the ligaments at their appropriate tensions, any other pair of surfaces that can fulfil that one function might be able to restore normal movements if all the ligaments are intact.

The evidence of the PTA and gait laboratory studies is that a spherical femoral condyle articulating on a flat tibial plateau can replace the natural surfaces of the medial com-partment. It is stressed that, in this regard, the meniscal bearing design of the OUKA implant is not different from fixed-bearing UKA implants, most of which employ a flat, or nearly flat, tibial plateau which allows the femoral condyle the same freedoms of anteroposterior translation as the OUKA enjoys. We know of no evidence, and there is no theoretical reason, for the biomechanics and kinematics of the two designs of implant to differ *as long as the tibial component of the fixed-bearing implant remains flat.*

However, if, because of the effects of wear, the flat form of the polyethylene becomes concave, the translational movements of the femoral condyle may become constrained. If stability can be restored to normal with the Oxford instrumentation it is likely to remain so because of the minimal wear of the meniscal bearing.

Mathematical models

Explanations for many of the above observations can be deduced from analysis of mathematical models of the knee. Two- and three-dimensional models are discussed in the Appendix, and animations of the models are available on the DVD provided with this book.

References

1. Taylor WR, Heller MO, Bergmann G, Duda GN. Tibio-femoral loading during normal daily activities. In: *Knee Arthroplasty: Engineering Functionality*. London: Institution of Mechanical Engineers, 2005; 142–5.
2. Rostoker W, Galante JO. Contact pressure dependence of wear rates of ultra high molecular weight polyethylene. *J Biomed Mater Res* 1979; **13**: 957–64.
3. Sathasivam S, Walker PS, Campbell PA, Rayner K. The effect of contact area on wear in relation to fixed bearing and mobile bearing knee replacements. *J Biomed Mater Res* 2001; **58**: 282–90.
4. Fairbank TJ. Knee joint changes after meniscectomy. *J Bone Joint Surg [Br]* 1948; **30-B**: 664–70.
5. Bullough PG, Munuera L, Murphy J, Weinstein AM. The strength of the menisci of the knee as it relates to their fine structure. *J Bone Joint Surg [Br]* 1970; **52-B**: 564–7.
6. Shrive NG, O'Connor JJ, Goodfellow JW. Load-bearing in the knee joint. *Clin Orthop* 1978; **131**: 279–87.
7. Borelli GA. *De Motu Animalium*, 1680. English translation by Maquet P. *On the movement of animals*. Heidelberg: Springer Verlag, 1989.
8. Kapandji I. *The Physiology of the Joints*. Vol II Edinburgh: Churchill Livingstone, 1970.
9. Thompson WO, Fu FH, Thaete FL, Dye S. Assessment of tibial meniscal kinematics by 3-D magnetic resonance imaging. *Trans Orthop Res Soc* 1990; **15**; 245.
10. Vedi V, Williams A, Tennant SJ, Spouse E, Hunt DM, Gedroyc WM. Meniscal movement. An *in-vivo* study using dynamic MRI. *J Bone Joint Surg [Br]* 1999; **81-B**: 37–41.
11. Goodfellow J, O'Connor J. The mechanics of the knee and prosthesis design. *J Bone Joint Surg [Br]* 1978; **60-B**: 358–69.
12. Buechel FF, Pappas MJ. The New Jersey Low-Contact-Stress Knee Replacement System: biomechanical rationale and review of the first 123 cemented cases. *Arch Orthop Trauma Surg* 1986; **105**: 197–204.
13. Argenson JN, O'Connor JJ. Polyethylene wear in meniscal knee replacement. A one to nine-year retrieval analysis of the Oxford Knee. *J Bone Joint Surg [Br]* 1992; **74-B**: 228–32.
14. Psychoyios V, Crawford RW, O'Connor JJ, Murray DW. Wear of congruent meniscal bearings in unicompartmental knee arthroplasty: a retrieval study of 16 specimens. *J Bone Joint Surg [Br]* 1998; **80-B**: 976–82.
15. Price AJ. Medial meniscal bearing unicompartmental arthroplasty: wear, mechanics and clinical outcome. DPhil Thesis, University of Oxford, 2003.
16. Short A, Gill HS, Marks B, Waite JC, Kellett CF, Price AJ, O'Connor JJ, Murray DW. A novel method for *in vivo* knee prosthesis wear measurement. *J Biomech* 2005; **38**: 315–22.

17. Price AJ, Short A, Kellett C, Beard D, Gill H, Dodd CAF, Murray DW. Ten year *in-vivo* wear measurement of a fully congruent mobile bearing unicompartmental knee arthroplasty. *J Bone Joint Surg [Br]* 2005; **87-B**: 1943–7.

18. Walker PS, Blunn GW, Broome DR, Perry J, Watkins A, Sathasivam S, Dewar ME, Paul JP. A knee simulating machine for performance evaluation of total knee replacements. *J Biomech* 1997; **30**: 83–9.

19. Scott R, Schroeder D. Correlation of knee simulator to *in-vivo* use: evaluating the Oxford Unicompartmental Knee. In: *Transactions of the 46th Annual Meeting of the Orthopaedic Research Society, 2000*, Orlando, Florida. Rosemont, IL: Orthopaedic Research Society, 2000; 434.

20. Morra EA, Greenwald AS. Effects of walking gait on ultra-high molecular weight polyethylene damage in unicompartmental knee systems. A finite element study. *J Bone Joint Surg [Am]* 2003; **85-A** (Suppl 4): 111–14.

21. Ashraf T, Newman JH, Desai VV, Beard D, Nevelos JE. Polyethylene wear in a non-congruous unicompartmental knee replacement: a retrieval analysis. *Knee* 2004; **11**: 177–81.

22. Wroblewski BM. Direction and rate of socket wear in Charnley low-friction arthroplasty. *J Bone Joint Surg [Br]* 1985; **67-B**: 757–61.

23. Plante-Bordeneuve P, Freeman MA. Tibial high-density polyethylene wear in conforming tibiofemoral prostheses. *J Bone Joint Surg [Br]* 1993; **75-B**: 630–6.

24. Hamelynck KJ, Stiehl JB, Voorhorst PE. Worldwide multicentre outcome study. In: Hamelynck KJ, Stiehl JB (ed). *LCS Mobile Bearing Arthroplasty. 25 Years of Worldwide Experience*. Berlin: Springer, 2002; 212–24.

25. Keblish PA, Briard JL. Mobile-bearing unicompartmental knee arthroplasty: a 2-center study with an 11-year (mean) follow-up. *J Arthroplasty* 2004; **19**(Suppl 2): 87–94.

26. Bartel DL, Bicknell VL, Wright TM. The effect of conformity, thickness, and material on stresses in ultra-high molecular weight components for total joint replacement. *J Bone Joint Surg [Am]* 1986; **68-A**: 1041–51.

27. Marmor L. The Modular (Marmor) knee: case report with a minimum follow-up of 2 years. *Clin Orthop* 1976; **120**: 86–94.

28. Kabo JM, Gebhard JS, Loren G, Amstutz HC. *In vivo* wear of polyethylene acetabular components. *J Bone Joint Surg [Br]* 1993; **75-B**: 254–8.

29. Hall RM, Siney P, Unsworth A, Wroblewski BM. The association between rates of wear in retrieved acetabular components and the radius of the femoral head. *J Engng Med, Proc Inst Mech Eng H* 1998; **212**: 321–6.

30. Wilson DR, Feikes JD, Zavatsky AB, O'Connor JJ. The components of passive knee movement are coupled to flexion angle. *J Biomech* 2000; **33**: 465–73.

31. Butler DL, Noyes FR, Grood ES. Ligamentous restraints to anterior–posterior drawer in the human knee. *J Bone Joint Surg [Am]* 1980; **62-A**: 259–70.

32. Grood ES, Noyes FR, Butler DL, Suntay WJ. Ligamentous and capsular restraints preventing straight medial and lateral laxity in intact human cadaver knees. *J Bone Joint Surg [Am]* 1981; **63-A**: 1257–69.

33. Piziali RL, Seering WP, Nagel DA, Schurman DJ. The function of the primary ligaments of the knee in anterior-posterior and medial-lateral motions. *J Biomech* 1980; **13**: 777–84.

34. Seering WP, Piziali RL, Nagel DA, Schurman DJ. The function of the primary ligaments of the knee in varus-valgus and axial rotation. *J Biomech* 1980; **13**: 785–94.

35. Feikes JD. The mobility and stability of the human knee joint. DPhil Thesis, University of Oxford, 1999.

36. Walker PS, Rovick JS, Robertson DD. The effects of knee brace hinge design and placement on joint mechanics. *J Biomech* 1988; **21**: 965–74.

37. Iwaki H, Pinskerova V, Freeman MA. Tibiofemoral movement. 1: The shapes and relative movements of the femur and tibia in the unloaded cadaver knee. *J Bone Joint Surg [Br]* 2000; **82-B**: 1189–95.

38. Rehder U. Morphometrical studies on the symmetry of the human knee joint: femoral condyles. *J Biomech* 1983; **16**: 351–61.

39. Bradley J, Goodfellow JW, O'Connor JJ. A radiographic study of bearing movement in unicompartmental Oxford Knee replacements. *J Bone Joint Surg [Br]* 1987; **69-B**: 598–601.

40. Kurosawa H, Walker PS, Abe S, Garg A, Hunter T. Geometry and motion of the knee for implant and orthotic design. *J Biomech* 1985; **18**: 487–99.

41. Miller RK, Goodfellow JW, Murray DW, O'Connor JJ. *In vitro* measurement of patellofemoral force after three types of knee replacement. *J Bone Joint Surg [Br]* 1998; **80-B**: 900–6.

42. Price AJ, Rees JL, Beard DJ, Gill RH, Dodd CA, Murray DM. Sagittal plane kinematics of a mobile-bearing unicompartmental knee arthroplasty at 10 years: a comparative *in vivo* fluoroscopic analysis. *J Arthroplasty* 2004; **19**: 590–7.

43. Jefferson RJ, Whittle MW. Biomechanical assessment of unicompartmental knee arthroplasty, total condylar arthroplasty and tibial osteotomy. *Clin Biomech* 1989; **4**: 232–42.

2

Indications

Total knee replacement is an effective treatment for most types of arthritis of the knee and requires little of the joint's anatomy to be intact for a successful outcome. However, unicompartmental arthroplasty can only succeed if the rest of the knee is functionally intact before surgery. We will discuss, first, the pathology of osteoarthritis (OA) of the knee and then how to ascertain, before operating, that the ligaments are all functionally normal and the retained articular surfaces capable of resuming their weight-bearing role.

History

The components of the OUKA prosthesis were first used (from 1976 to 1984) as a bi-compartmental knee replacement (Fig. 2.1). The patients had severe OA or rheumatoid arthritis and since, at that time, there were no proven alternative treatments, there were no specific indications. The first step towards defining a role for the implant was taken when the results of these operations were reviewed and it was found that the anatomical state of the anterior cruciate ligament (ACL) at the time of surgery was an important determinant of the long-term outcome [1]. In 1992, we reported a six-fold difference in the 7-year cumulative survival of the prosthesis between knees with or without a functioning ACL at the time of surgery, irrespective of the primary disease and of all the other variables measured [2]. This was the first publication to offer statistical evidence of the importance of that ligament in the kinematics of unconstrained resurfacing implants. During the same period we had, incidentally, observed that in osteoarthritic knees with an intact ACL, articular surface damage was usually limited to the medial compartment, with the rest of the joint remaining healthy. Taken together, the two observations suggest-

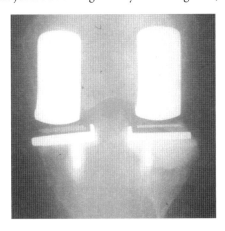

Figure 2.1 Bicompartmental Oxford Knee replacement (Phase 1).

ed that these cases would be appropriate for treatment with the meniscal prosthesis and, since 1982, the implant has been mainly used for medial replacement in OA knees with intact ACL [3].

Subsequently, we published a more detailed study of the pattern of cartilage damage in arthritis, correlating the preoperative clinical and radiological signs with the intraoperative findings during unicompartmental surgery [4]. In that paper we introduced the term 'anteromedial osteoarthritis' to describe the subgroup of varus knees in which both cruciate ligaments and the MCL are functionally normal, and in which the cartilage and bone erosions are in the anterior and central parts of the medial compartment.

We now believe that anteromedial OA is the most common indication for UKA. The syndrome can be recognized by a consistent association between the clinical and radio-logical signs and the pathological lesions that cause them.

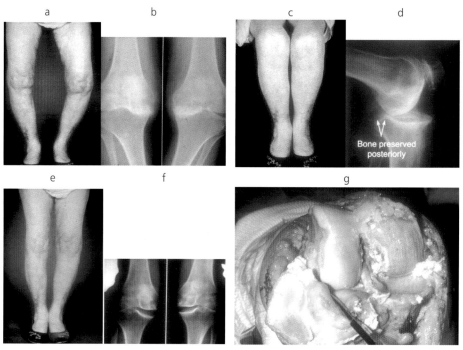

Figure 2.2 The patient illustrated had unusually severe bilateral anteromedial OA. Standing, (a) she has marked varus deformities and the radiographs (b) show deep erosions of both medial tibial plateaux. Sitting, (c) the varus corrects. The radiograph (d) shows that this is because the medial condyles roll out of the anteromedial erosions on to the intact articular surfaces posteriorly. Because the varus corrected every time the knees were flexed, structural shortening of the medial collateral ligament could not occur. Therefore, with the knees flexed a little, the patient could correct the varus with her own muscles (e). On the radiographs (f), the varus is corrected by applied valgus force. The intraoperative picture shows the anatomical features of anteromedial OA. Note the intact ACL. (Reproduced with permission and copyright © of the British Editorial Society of Bone and Joint Surgery [White SH, Ludkowski PF, Goodfellow JW. Anteromedial osteoarthritis of the knee. *J Bone Joint Surg [Br]* 1991; **73-B**: 582–6].)

Anteromedial osteoarthritis (Fig. 2.2)

Principal physical signs

1. Pain in the knee is present on standing and is severe when walking. It is relieved by sitting.
2. With the knee (as near as possible) fully extended, the leg is in varus (5–15°) and the deformity cannot be corrected.
3. With the knee flexed 20° or more, the varus can be corrected.
4. With the knee flexed to 90°, the varus corrects spontaneously.

Principal anatomical features

At surgery, knees with the above physical signs regularly demonstrate the following anatomical features, some of which are visible in the intraoperative photograph shown in Figure 2.2 and all of which are illustrated in the diagrams in Figure 2.3.

1. Both cruciate ligaments are functionally normal, though the ACL may have suffered surface damage.
2. The cartilage on the tibia is eroded, and eburnated bone is exposed, in an area that extends from the anteromedial margin of the medial plateau for a variable distance posteriorly but never as far as the posterior margin. An area of full-thickness cartilage is always preserved at the back of the plateau (Fig. 2.3(a)).
3. The cartilage on the inferior articular surface of the medial femoral condyle is eroded, and eburnated bone is exposed. The posterior surface of the condyle retains its full-thickness cartilage (Fig. 2.3(a)).
4. The articular cartilage of the lateral compartment, although often fibrillated, preserves its full thickness (Fig. 2.3(b)).
5. The medial collateral ligament (MCL) is of normal length (Fig. 2.3(d) and Fig. 2.3(f)).
6. The posterior capsule is shortened (Fig. 2.3(a)).

Correlations

The observed sites of articular surface damage, together with the intact status of the cruciate ligaments and the MCL, explain the symptoms and physical signs.

1. The cruciate ligaments maintain the normal pattern of 'rollback' of the femur on the tibia in the sagittal plane and thereby preserve the distinction between the damaged contact areas in extension (the anterior tibial plateau and the inferior surface of the medial femoral condyle) (Figs. 2.3(a) and (b)) and the intact contact areas in flexion (the posterior tibial plateau and the posterior surface of the femoral condyle). (Figs. 2.3(c) and (d)). The short posterior capsule causes the flexion deformity (Fig. 2.3(a)).
2. The varus deformity of the extended leg, (and the pain felt on standing and walking), are caused by loss of cartilage and bone from the contact areas in extension (Figs. 2.3(a) and 2.3(b)).

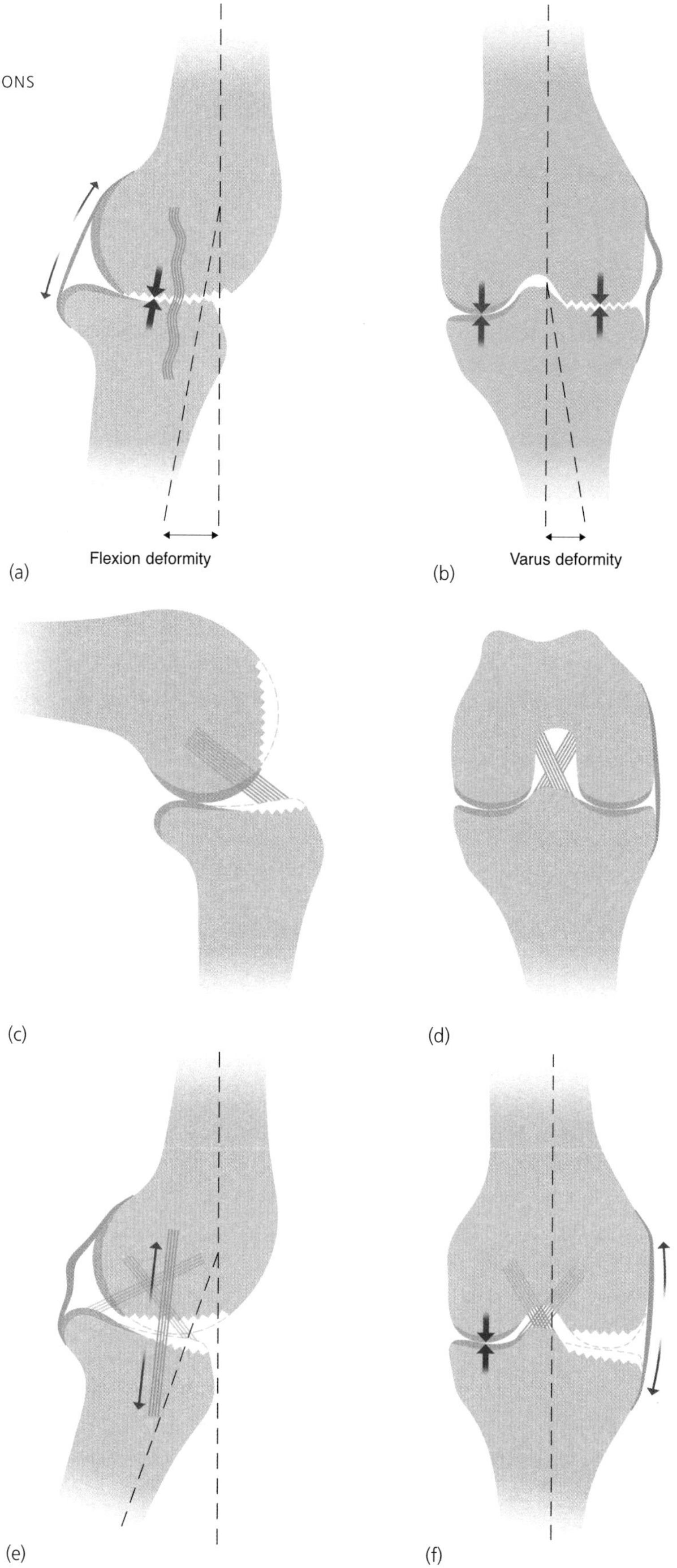

Figure 2.3 Diagramatic explanation of the physical signs of anteromedial OA (see text).

The *angle* of varus depends on the amount of material lost. To expose bone on both surfaces, the total thickness of cartilage lost is about 5 mm, causing about 5° of varus. At least this degree of deformity is usual on presentation because pain seldom becomes severe until there is bone-on-bone contact during weight bearing. Thereafter, each millimetre of bone eroded increases the deformity by about 1°.

3. The varus deformity corrects spontaneously at 90° as the cartilage is intact in the areas of contact in flexion (Figs. 2.3(c) and 2.3(d)). Therefore the MCL is drawn out to its normal length every time the patient bends the knee (Fig. 2.3(d)), and structural shortening of the ligament does not occur. Thus an intact ACL ensures an MCL of normal length, as demonstrated by manual correction of the varus (Fig. 2.3(f)) when the posterior capsule is relaxed (Figs. 2.3(e)) by flexing the knee 20°.

Progression to posteromedial osteoarthritis

The association of an intact ACL with the focal pattern of cartilage erosions described above is striking. White *et al.* [4] described 46 medial tibial plateaux excised sequentially from a series of OA knees treated by OUKA, all of them with an intact ACL and with car-

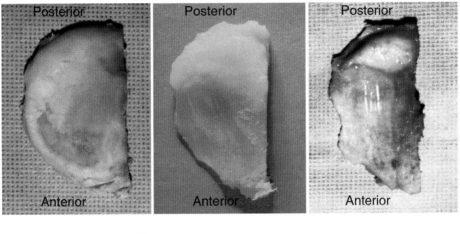

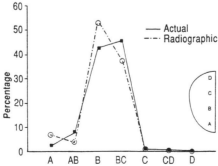

Figure 2.4 Typical tibial plateau lesions of anteromedial OA. The graph compares radiographic data with data from 46 intraoperative specimens. (The graph is reproduced with permission and copyright © of the British Editorial Society of Bone and Joint Surgery [White SH, Ludkowski PF, Goodfellow JW. Anteromedial osteoarthritis of the knee. *J Bone Joint Surg [Br]* 1991; **73-B**: 582–6].)

tilage erosions exposing bone (Ahlback stages 2, 3, and 4). The erosions were *all* anterior and central (Fig. 2.4). They rarely extended to the posterior quarter of the plateau and *never* reached the posterior joint margin.

Harman *et al.* [5] examined the tibial plateaux excised from 143 osteoarthritic knees during operations for TKA. They found that wear in ACL-deficient varus knees was located a mean 4 mm more posterior on the medial plateau than wear in ACL-intact knees ($P < 0.05$). The ACL-deficient knees also exhibited more severe varus deformity. The authors stated: '… it is evident that anterior cruciate ligament integrity is a dominant factor affecting the location of tibiofemoral contact and the resulting cartilage wear patterns in patients with osteoarthritis'.

The site and extent of the tibial erosions can be reliably determined from lateral radiographs (see Fig. 2.4) [4]. Based on this, Keys *et al.* [6] studied the preoperative lateral radiographs of 50 OA knees in which the state of the ACL had been recorded at surgery (25 ACL deficient and 25 ACL intact). Using four blinded observers, they found 95 per cent correlation between preservation of the posterior part of the medial tibial plateau on the radiograph and an intact ACL at surgery, and 100 per cent correlation of erosion of the posterior plateau on the radiograph with an absent or badly damaged ACL.

These correlations show that, as long as the ACL remains intact, the tibiofemoral contact areas in flexion remain distinct from the areas of contact in extension. Progressive loss of bone causes the varus deformity in extension to increase but, while the ACL continues to function, the deformity corrects spontaneously in flexion and structural shortening of the MCL does not occur.

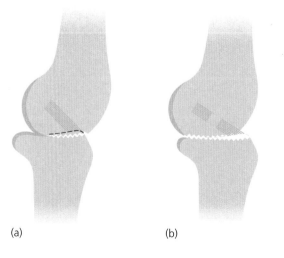

(a)   (b)

Figure 2.5 (a) The intact ACL holds the femur forward on the tibia in extension. (b) Rupture (or stretching) of the ACL allows posterior subluxation of the femur on the tibia and secondary damage to the posterior articular surface of the tibial plateau. (Thereafter the cartilage on the posterior surface of the femur is damaged when the femur flexes.)

Failure of the ACL may be the event that causes the transition from anteromedial OA to the posteromedial form of the disease, with posterior subluxation of the femur and structural shortening of the MCL. Deschamps and Lapeyre [7] observed that absence of the ACL in an osteoarthritic knee was associated with posterior subluxation of the femur on the tibia in extension. Figure 2.5 demonstrates how this subluxation results in abrasion of the cartilage at the back of the tibial plateau by the exposed bone on the inferior surface of the femoral condyle. Thereafter, in flexion, the cartilage on the posterior surface of the femoral condyle is also destroyed by abrasion on the tibial plateau, now devoid of cartilage. The varus deformity is then present in flexion as well as in extension, and the MCL can shorten structurally.

The sequence described above does not require us to assume any 'spread' of the original disease to adjacent intact cartilage. Failure of the ACL alone is enough to explain how the original lesions in the 'extension areas' of the medial compartment could cause secondary physical damage to the cartilage of its 'flexion areas' and start a process that results in a subluxed knee with progressive bone loss posteromedially and fixed varus deformity.

How and why does the ACL rupture?

How?

The stages of deterioration observed intraoperatively in OA knees suggest the following sequence:

- normal
- loss of synovial covering, usually starting distally
- longitudinal splits in the substance of the exposed ligament
- stretching and loss of strength of the collagen bundles
- rupture and eventual disappearance of the ligament.

Why?

Among the knee's ligaments, the ACL is peculiarly at risk because of two anatomical features.

1. Its intra-articular course puts it at risk of nutritional insufficiency from chronic synovitis of any type. For instance, the ACL is frequently damaged by chronic rheumatoid synovitis. The importance of the ligament's synovial investment is also suggested by the observation that the ACL is always healthy in knees in which the ligamentum mucosum is intact (Dr RD Scott, personal communication). Experimental stripping of the synovium from rabbit ACL causes a succession of changes very like those seen in human OA joints, culminating in structural disintegration of the ligament [8].

2. The ligament is at risk of physical damage from osteophytes at the margins of the condyles. In knees with anteromedial OA, osteophytes are almost always present on the lateral side, and sometimes on both sides of the intercondylar notch, and the lower part of the ligament may be damaged by them as the knee approaches full extension (Fig. 2.6).

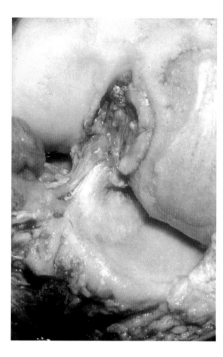

Figure 2.6 Intraoperative picture of an ACL surrounded by osteophytes and partly denuded of its synovium.

Chronic synovitis and osteophytosis, which are both common in antereomedial OA, probably represent the response throughout the joint cavity to material shed into it from the cartilage erosions in the medial compartment.

Summary of pathology

The primary pathological lesions of anteromedial OA are focal erosions of the cartilage on the inferior surface of the medial femoral condyle and on the anterior and central parts of the medial tibial plateau, areas that make contact with one another in extension.

Chronic synovitis and marginal osteophytosis are secondary pathological changes. The articular cartilage of the lateral compartment is functionally intact. The cruciate and collateral ligaments are of normal length.

While the ACL remains effective, the orderly flexion–extension movements of the femur on the tibia in the sagittal plane are preserved, maintaining the separation of the flexion areas from the extension areas. Progressive loss of bone causes increasing varus deformity in extension but not in flexion.

Failure of the ACL allows posterior subluxation of the femur on the tibia and offers a sufficient explanation for the progression from anteromedial arthritis to posteromedial disease.

If this is the natural history, resurfacing the medial compartment *while the ACL is still intact* may cure the symptoms and recover the normal kinematics and mechanics of the joint. If the osteophytes have been removed, and cartilage debris is no longer shed into the joint cavity, later failure of the ACL and spread of the disease to the other compartments may be avoided.

These are the theoretical reasons for employing unicompartmental arthroplasty as the treatment for anteromedial OA.

Preoperative assessment

Preoperative assessment aims to determine, as precisely as possible, whether a particular knee has anteromedial OA.

Clinical examination

Pain

Pain is usually felt near the medial joint line but it may be anterior, posterior, and even on the lateral side of the knee. Its localization is not a reliable sign. Pain is felt on standing and walking, but is usually absent while sitting (when the intact articular surfaces at the back of the medial compartment are in contact) and when lying down (when the damaged surfaces are unloaded).

Severity of pain and limitation of walking distance are the factors that decide the need for operation. The criteria are similar to those used to justify TKA.

Physical signs

The principal physical signs were briefly described in the previous section.

1. Varus deformity of the leg is best seen when the patient is standing. Varus is seldom less than 5° on presentation and rarely more than 15°. Greater deformity than this is usually associated with failure of the ACL and therefore is a contraindication. A 'lateral thrust' of the knee is often seen on walking and is not a contraindication.

   As already noted, the varus deformity corrects spontaneously when the patient is seated with the knee flexed to 90° (see Fig. 2.3(c) and (d)), and it can be manually corrected, by applying a valgus force, with the knee flexed 20° or more to relax the posterior capsule (see Fig. 2.3(e) and (f)).

2. Usually the knee will not fully extend but flexion deformity is seldom more than 10°. More than 15° is a contraindication. Flexion deformity persists under anaesthesia and is due to structural shortening of the posterior capsule and/or the presence of osteophytes (see below).

3. Flexion range is usually limited but is rarely less than 100°. Severe limitation of flexion is a relative contraindication to OUKA because of the difficulty it presents at surgery. However, more flexion can usually be achieved under anaesthesia than in the clinic, particularly if the limitation is due to severe pain rather than stiffness of the joint.

4. Moderate synovial swelling and joint effusion are common, and there is often tenderness to palpation over the medial joint line.

It should be noted that the 'pivot shift', the drawer test, and other manoeuvres designed to assess the cruciate ligaments after trauma are of much less value in the arthritic knee. Erroneous conclusions may result from false instability, due to intact ligaments being rendered slack by loss of articular cartilage height, or from false stability, due to interpenetration of the damaged articular surfaces, or the presence of large osteophytes, which mask ligament insufficiency. These tests are not used in preoperative decision-making.

Radiography

Radiography is the most useful adjunct to physical signs in demonstrating the suitability of a knee for OUKA.

Anteroposterior radiographs

Anteroposterior radiographs, taken in the standard way with the patient weight-bearing on the extended leg, can demonstrate loss of articular cartilage medially by showing that the condyles articulate 'bone-on-bone' (Ahlback stage 2 or more). However, in some cases in which there is full-thickness cartilage loss, this method fails to reveal it. A better projection for this purpose is with the patient standing with the knee 15° flexed, with the X-ray beam appropriately tilted. A non-weight-bearing varus-stressed film is more reliable than either of these methods (Fig. 2.7).

Valgus-stressed radiographs

Valgus-stressed radiographs are used to ensure that there is a normal thickness of articular cartilage in the lateral compartment and to demonstrate that the intra articular varus deformity is correctable (i.e. the MCL is not shortened). We have found no other

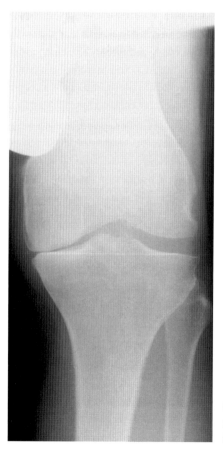

Figure 2.7 Varus stressed radiograph of anteromedial OA.

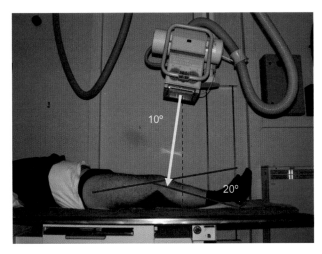

Figure 2.8 Technique of varus/valgus stress radiography.

method of investigation to be so satisfactory in confirming these two key requirements for successful unicompartmental replacement [9].

When the patient stands on a knee with a varus deformity, body weight tends to distract the lateral joint surfaces [10,11]. Therefore, to measure the thickness of the lateral compartment cartilage, the lateral condyles must be firmly apposed to one another by applying a valgus force to the otherwise unloaded limb.

Technique (Fig. 2.8)

The patient lies supine on the X-ray couch with a support under the knee to flex it 20°. The X-ray beam is aligned 10° from the vertical (to allow for the average posterior inclination of the tibial plateau). The surgeon (wearing protective gloves and apron) applies a firm valgus couple of forces through the knee, ensuring that the leg is in neutral rotation.

Interpretation (Fig. 2.9)

1. The radiolucent joint space between the subchondral plates of the lateral compartment should measure not less than 5 mm, the sum of the thickness of two layers of normal cartilage (Fig. 2.9(b)). Narrowing of the gap implies thinning of the cartilage and its impending failure. It is a contraindication to UKA.

2. If the damaged medial condyles have separated to reveal a radiolucent gap of at least 5 mm (previously occupied by articular cartilage), the genu varum is fully correctable and the MCL is not shortened. This gap may be greater than 5 mm, depending on how much bone, as well as cartilage, has been lost (see Fig. 2.2(f)).

(We do not attempt to assess the overall alignment of the leg on stress radiographs as small degrees of rotation can give a false impression.)

Varus-stressed radiographs

Varus-stressed radiographs are the most reliable radiographic method for demonstrating full-thickness loss of cartilage (bone-on-bone contact) between the medial condyles (see Fig. 2.9(a)). As mentioned above, the commonly employed weight-bearing projections

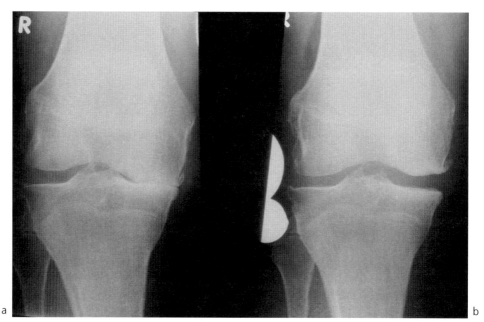

a   b

Figure 2.9 Varus/valgus stress radiographs

are often adequate, and if they are available and positive there is no need of further evidence. Similarly, if eburnated bone has been seen arthroscopically on both surfaces, no further evidence is required. However, if there is doubt, it is best resolved by employing the technique described above, but with a varus force applied (see Fig. 2.9(a)).

Failure to demonstrate bone-on-bone contact by this method is, we believe, a contraindication to joint replacement. Mere thinning of the cartilage and surface fibrillation with marginal osteophytes (Ahlback stage 1) is a dubious explanation for disabling pain. If eburnated bone-on-bone contact cannot be demonstrated, other causes for the pain should be looked for.

Lateral radiographs

The lateral radiograph demonstrates the site and posterior extent of any bone erosion on the tibial plateau. It is a reliable indicator of the functional integrity of the ACL and therefore of the suitability of the knee for OUKA.

Technique The patient lies on his or her side on the X-ray couch, with the knee flexed 20°. The outer side of the knee is in contact with the plate and the X-ray source is about 1 m distant.

Interpretation The femoral condyles and the tibial plateaux should appear superimposed. If they are not, the radiograph is difficult to interpret and should be repeated. The tibial plateaux can be distinguished from one another by the different shapes of their posterior margins as described by Jacobsen [12] (Fig. 2.10). Sclerosis of the subchondral bone medially makes this distinction more obvious in the arthritic than in the normal knee.

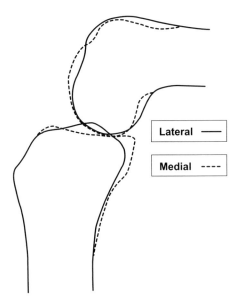

Lateral ———

Medial ----

Figure 2.10 The distinctive profiles of the posterior margins of the medial and lateral tibial plateaux. (After K. Jacobsen, *Acta Orthop Scand Suppl* 1981; **194**: 1–263.)

1. If there is no bone erosion visible (Ahlback stage 2), the ACL is almost certainly intact.
2. When there is bone erosion (Ahlback stages 3 and 4), a concave defect is seen. If the greatest depth of the concavity is in the anterior half of the plateau or central, and the erosion does not extend to the posterior margin of the plateau, the ACL is intact (95 per cent probability) (Fig. 2.11, and compare with Fig. 2.4).
3. If the bone erosion extends to the back of the plateau, or if there is posterior subluxation of the femur, the ACL is almost certainly absent or severely damaged [6] and OUKA is not appropriate (Fig. 2.11).

It should be noted that while MRI is useful for diagnosing traumatic lesions of the ACL, it has been found to have little value in characterizing the functional integrity of the ligament in degenerative disease [13]. Nor do we regularly employ preoperative arthroscopy, having found the radiographic evidence of the posterior extent of the tibial erosion a more reliable (if indirect) measure of the ligament's functional efficacy.

Other radiographic observations

Osteophytes Osteophytes are commonly seen at the margins of all the articular surfaces. Their presence around the lateral and patellofemoral surfaces does not indicate damage to the weight-bearing areas of these compartments. The presence of osteophytes at certain sites should be noted so that they can be removed at surgery.

On the lateral projection, there is often an osteophyte on the posterior margin of the medial tibial plateau which makes delivery of the plateau difficult (Fig. 2.12). Those on the back of the medial femoral condyle are sometimes large and may contribute to the flexion deformity by 'tenting' the posterior capsule. They can also impinge against the bearing in full flexion.

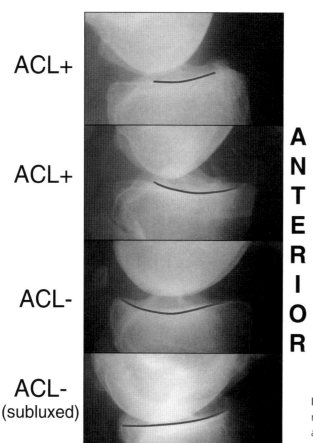

ACL+

ACL+

ACL-

ACL-
(subluxed)

A
N
T
E
R
I
O
R

Figure 2.11 Series of lateral radiographs of knees with anteromedial OA to show various depths and posterior extents of the tibial erosions.

An osteophyte may be seen arising from the intercondylar region of the tibia, anterior to the attachment of the ACL. It can impinge against the femur in extension and constitute a block to the recovery of full extension.

Mediolateral subluxation When there is significant loss of bone from the medial compartment (varus greater than 10°), the AP standing and the varus-stressed films may show lateral subluxation of the femur on the tibia (Fig. 2.13). If the valgus-stressed film shows complete reduction of the subluxation and the varus, both will be corrected by the operation and the subluxation can be ignored. If the subluxation persists on the valgus-stressed film, it is a contraindication to OUKA.

Intraoperative observations

The clinical and radiographic examinations described above can predict the suitability of a knee for Oxford arthroplasty with an accuracy of better than 90 per cent. However, the final decision, whether to proceed with unicompartmental or total replacement, is best taken on the operating table when the joint has been opened.

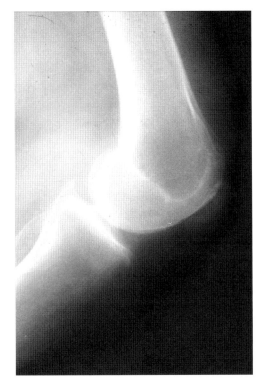

Figure 2.12 Radiograph of posterior tibial osteophyte.

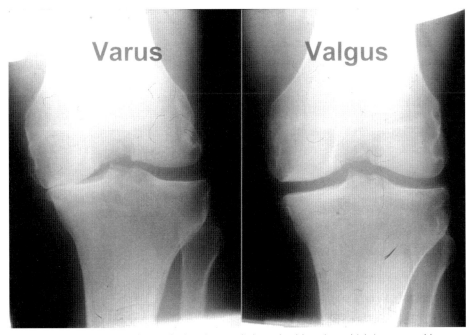

Figure 2.13 Varus stress radiograph showing mediolateral subluxation which is corrected by valgus stress.

ACL damage Direct examination of the ACL may cause a change of mind. ACL deterioration is gradual (as is the posterior extension of the tibial erosion), and it is sometimes difficult to determine the point at which the ACL has ceased to function adequately.

To increase the precision of the indications, we analysed retrospectively two large series of OUKAs in which the state of the ACL had been recorded intraoperatively [14,15]. The subjects were all followed for at least 10 years with no significant loss to follow-up. The 10-year cumulative survival for knees in which the synovial lining was partly missing, and for those with longitudinal splits in the ligament's substance, was the same as for knees with 'normal' ligaments, i.e. intact synovial investment. On the basis of this study, we recommend the following.

- Loss of synovial lining, even if it is accompanied by longitudinal splits in the substance of the ligament, is not a contraindication.
- Knees in which the ligament is ruptured or its substance is demonstrably weak are unsuitable for OUKA.

A practical way to show that a ligament is 'demonstrably weak' is to insert a small hook into its substance (through a longitudinal split) and pull forcibly on a bundle of fibres. If they do not rupture, it is safe to proceed to OUKA; if they rupture, TKA is required.

Lateral compartment damage Even through the small incision now used for OUKA, it is possible to see most of the articular surface of the lateral femoral condyle. Surface flaking and chondromalacia are very common and have been shown not to be significant. Occasionally, however, a full-thickness defect in the weight-bearing cartilage is discovered that has escaped radiographic detection. We treat this as a contraindication (although we have no evidence to support this practice).

It is important to know that when there is a significant varus deformity, there is often a circumscribed area of cartilage erosion (which can be up to 1 cm wide and 2 cm long) on the medial margin of the lateral femoral condyle, with eburnated bone exposed in its floor (see Fig. 2.6). This erosion may be a consequence of the varus alignment causing the margin of the femoral condyle to impinge on the tibial eminence. Impingement no longer occurs when the varus is corrected, as can be verified at the end of the operation. We do not consider this common lesion on the articular margin to be a contraindication to OUKA.

Summary of indications

The indications for OUKA in osteoarthritis are as follows.

Physical signs

1. Pain severe enough to justify joint replacement.
2. Flexion deformity less than 15°.

Radiographic signs

3. Full-thickness cartilage loss with eburnated bone-on-bone contact in the medial compartment (Ahlback stage 2, 3, or 4).

4. Full-thickness cartilage preserved in the lateral compartment.

5. Intact articular surface at the back of the tibial plateau.

6. Intra articular varus deformity manually correctable (in 20° flexion).

Intraoperative signs

7. Presence of an intact ACL (ignoring synovial damage and longitudinal splits).

8. Satisfactory appearance of the central articular cartilage of the lateral compartment.

Apart from the severity of the pain, all the indications that a knee is suitable for OUKA are anatomical. Plain radiography and stressed films are the best ways to demonstrate them.

Discussion of indications

In this section, some of the criteria listed above are discussed in more detail.

Flexion deformity

There may be several contributory causes for the (usually small) flexion deformity commonly seen in knees with anteromedial OA.

1. The posterior capsule is structurally shortened, perhaps from the effect of chronic synovitis and/or the patient's prolonged reluctance to straighten the painful knee.

2. Osteophytes at the posterior margin of the medial femoral condyle can 'tent' the posterior capsular ligament.

3. Osteophytes in the intercondylar notch of the femur can impinge, near full extension, on an osteophyte arising from the tibia in front of the attachment of the ACL.

It seems likely that there is always some structural shortening of the posterior capsule because removal of the osteophytes at surgery, although it often improves the deformity, does not immediately restore full extension. However, unlike TKA, unicompartmental replacement is followed in the postoperative period by spontaneous improvement of extension, probably from stretching of the shortened posterior capsule.

Weale *et al.* [16] reported that 28 knees with a mean preoperative flexion deformity of 8° (SD 8) reduced to a mean of 1° (SD 2) 1–2 years after OUKA ($P < 0.001$). At 10+ years, the mean deformity was not significantly changed (3° (SD 4)).

Provided that anterior and posterior osteophytes are removed, some correction will occur during the operation and improvement will continue in the succeeding year, so that a preoperative flexion deformity of as much as 15° is considered acceptable. In fact, it is unusual to encounter as great a deformity as this in an OA knee with an intact ACL. However, in avascular necrosis (AVN), with severe collapse of the femoral condyle, greater degrees of flexion deformity are encountered and have been found to correct spontaneously after OUKA.

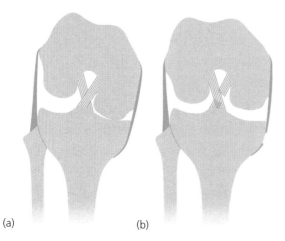

(a)   (b)

Figure 2.14 (a) In the normal knee in 90° flexion, the LCL allows about 6 mm distraction of the lateral compartment (see Fig 2.1(b)). (b) In TKA, the ACL is absent (or excised) and the MCL is lengthened surgically to match the LCL. The 'quadrilateral' flexion gap created is, then, wider than normal.

Why does flexion deformity correct spontaneously after UKA and not after TKA?

In TKA, 'balancing the ligaments' in flexion means equalizing the lengths of the MCL and the lateral collateral ligament (LCL) to create a quadrilateral flexion gap (Fig. 2.14). This is achieved by lengthening the MCL (Fig 2.14(b)), which leaves the flexion gap wider than before and the posterior capsule relatively too short. Therefore spontaneous correction of residual flexion deformity after TKA would require the posterior capsule to stretch beyond its physiological length.

In UKA, the cruciate mechanism and the MCL are both preserved intact and the flexion gap is the same after the operation as before, so that the posterior capsule is required only to stretch back to its physiological length for the flexion deformity to correct. Alteration of the interstriational angle of the lattice-like structure of the posterior capsule provides a mechanism whereby it could shorten, and lengthen again, but only within the limit set by the physiological lengths of its constituent fibres (Fig. 2.15).

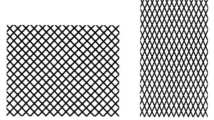

Figure 2.15 The posterior capsule's ability to shorten, and lengthen again, may be explained by the lattice-like arrangement of its collagen bundles.

Full-thickness cartilage in the lateral compartment

The full thickness of the cartilage is taken to be evidence that it is adequate to sustain load even if its surface is fibrillated and has superficial erosions.

Fibrillation and chondromalacia are almost always present in parts of the lateral (and patellofemoral) compartments of knees with anteromedial OA, probably because of the chronic synovitis present throughout the joint cavity and the abnormal loading regime

Table 2.1 Radiological evaluation of the lateral tibiofemoral compartment 10+ years after OUKA compared with its status at one year

Condition	Ahlback classification		Altman classification	
	Reading 1	Reading 2	Reading 1	Reading 2
Definitely worse	0	0	1	1
Possibly worse	7	3	5	6
Same	14	19	14	13
Possibly better	2	1	3	3
Definitely better	0	0	0	0

(The table is reproduced with permission and copyright © of the British Editorial Society of Bone and Joint Surgery [Weale AE, Murray DW, Crawford R, Psychoyios V, Bonomo A, Howell G, O'Connor J, Goodfellow JW. Does arthritis progress in the retained compartments after 'Oxford' medical unicompartmental arthroplasty? *J Bone Joint Surg [Br]* 1999; **81-B**: 783–9].)

experienced by the cartilage as a result of the varus deformity. It is because surface changes have proved largely irrelevant in predicting long-term outcome that arthroscopy does not appear among the necessary preoperative investigations listed above.

However, thinning of the articular cartilage in the lateral compartment is taken to be a sign of its impending failure to support load and is a contraindication to UKA. Therefore accurate measurement of cartilage thickness is important. We have tried ultrasound imaging and MRI, but have found these methods less reliable than the valgus-stressed plain radiograph (which has the added advantage of showing, at the same time, whether the varus is correctable).

The justification for the advice given above rests mainly on several published 10-year survival studies for OUKA performed using these criteria. In one study [16] there was no radiological evidence of deterioration during that time. Table 2.1 compares the appearance of the lateral compartment on radiographs taken immediately postoperatively with its appearance 10+ years later (mean interval 11.4 years). The films were all taken under fluoroscopic control and therefore were strictly comparable. The intra-observer error was small ($K = 0.64$) for the Ahlback classification and moderate ($K = 0.44$) for the Altman grading [17,18]. One lateral compartment in 23 knees examined showed definite progression of arthritis, but only on the Altman classification. Statistical analysis of the scores revealed no significant deterioration with time.

Nevertheless, failure of the lateral compartment has been a cause for revision of OUKA (see Chapter 6). The question as to whether the failure rate from this cause could be diminished by employing different, or more stringent, preoperative criteria than those advised above will only be answered by further prospective long-term studies. This matter is discussed in Chapter 6 where it is concluded that many lateral compartment failures result from overloading of the cartilage by inadvertent overcorrection into valgus, not from spontaneous degeneration with time.

Correctable varus deformity

Why do we not include full-length leg films in our preoperative radiological assessment?

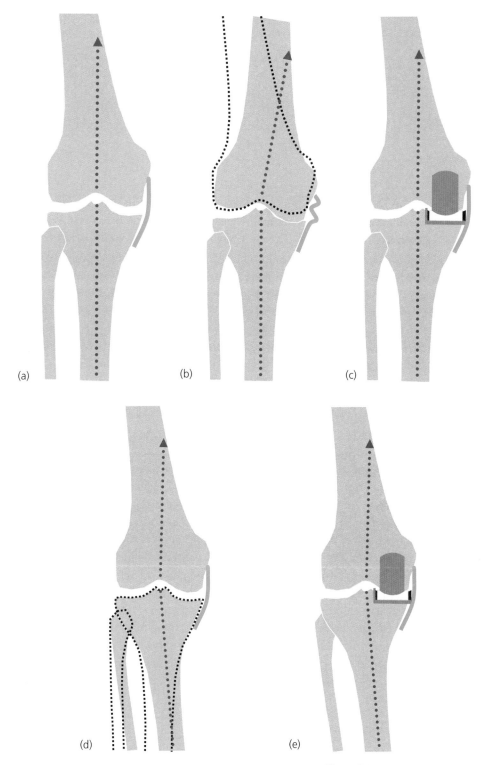

(a)

(b)

(c)

(d)

(e)

Figure 2.16 Genu varum and tibia vara (see text).

Tibiofemoral varus may be due to intra-articular deformity (genu varum) (Fig. 2.16(b)), extra-articular deformity (tibia vara) (Fig. 2.16(d)), or a combination of both.

1. The genu varum of anteromedial OA is caused by collapse of the medial compartment from loss of its cartilage and subchondral bone. The MCL is not shortened and so varus is completely correctable preoperatively, and completely corrected by OUKA. If the tibiofemoral angle was normal before the onset of arthritis (Fig. 2.16(a)), it will be returned to normal by the operation (Fig. 2.16(c)).

2. Tibia vara is a bone deformity, usually between the tibial plateau and the shaft (Fig. 2.16(d)), and is commonly developmental.

3. Not uncommonly, anteromedial OA develops in a limb with pre-existing extra-articular tibia vara, resulting in an increase in the tibiofemoral varus. In these cases, OUKA corrects the intra-articular genu varum but the tibia vara persists (Fig. 2.16(e)), so that the tibiofemoral angle remains in some degree of varus. (Much less commonly, genu varum develops in a limb with extra-articular *valgus*, which may be in the femur or the tibia. In this case, OUKA corrects the genu varum and restores whatever degree of tibiofemoral valgus was present before the arthritis developed.)

Therefore the term 'fully correctable' refers only to the intra-articular component of alignment deformity. The valgus-stressed radiograph predicts full correction of the intra-articular deformity by demonstrating at least 5 mm separation of the medial femoral condyle from the tibial plateau, i.e. the MCL is not shortened (see Fig. 2.9).

Measurement of the tibiofemoral shaft angle does not distinguish between intra-articular and extra-articular deformity and therefore is not helpful.

Emerson *et al.* [19] compared the effects on postoperative leg alignment of employing either a fixed-bearing UKA (Brigham) or an OUKA (Phase 2). They measured alignment on 3-foot anteroposterior radiographs taken with the patient standing. The technique of Kennedy and White [20] was used to determine the location in the knee through which the mechanical axis passed, and the conventions of the Knee Society to measure the angle of alignment. The average preoperative alignment of the two groups was similar, 1.7° and 1.8° varus. After OUKA the average alignment was 5.5° valgus, and after the fixed-bearing UKA it was 2.6° valgus. The variability of alignment after OUKA was less. Figure 2.17 shows that after OUKA the mechanical axis of the limb usually passed through the intercondylar area of the knee. The authors suggested that the greater degree of valgus achieved by the OUKA might explain the late failures from lateral compartment arthritis that they experienced.

Hernigou and Deschamps [21] showed that, after medial UKA, 'severe undercorrection' (i.e. hip–knee–ankle angle <170°) caused increased polyethylene wear in the fixed-bearing implants they used; and overcorrection into valgus (>180°) was associated with an increased risk of lateral compartment arthritis. However, their method of measurement could not distinguish between intra- and extra-articular deformity. Intra-articular overcorrection, implying as it does a damaged MCL, has been associated with lateral compartment arthritis after OUKA. However, failure of a meniscal bearing from wear-through has not been recorded, although some limbs have residual extra-articular varus.

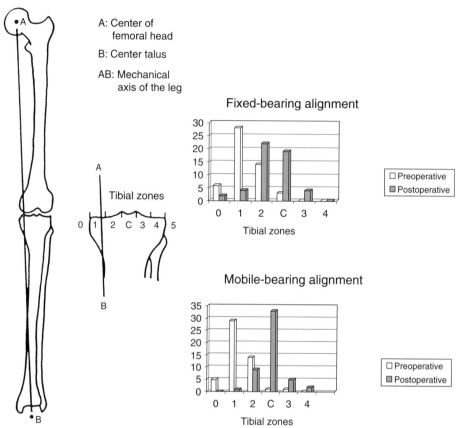

Figure 2.17 The mechanical axis of the leg is shown with the tibial surface divided into zones. The zone location of the mechanical axis for the fixed- and mobile-bearing knee implants taken with 3-foot radiographs obtained with the patient standing are shown in graphical form. The tibial zones are according to Kennedy and White [20]. (Reproduced with permission of Lippincott Williams & Wilkins from Emerson RH Jr., Hansborough T, Reitman RD, Rosenfeldt W, Higgins LL. Comparison of a mobile with a fixed-bearing unicompartmental knee implant. *Clin Orthop* 2002; **404**: 62–70.)

We believe that no attempt should ever be made to correct an extra-articular varus malalignment intra-articularly (e.g. by MCL release). On the contrary, that ligament's fibres should all be carefully preserved, and 'overstuffing' of the medial compartment with a bearing that is too thick should be avoided.

Not contraindications

While it is important to ensure that all the necessary indications are met, it is also important not to apply unnecessary contraindications. Some published lists of supposed contra-indications have achieved wide acceptance without having much evidence to support them.

Age

Old age has been proposed as a relative contraindication [22]. In our opinion, the lower morbidity and quicker recovery of UKA recommend it in all elderly subjects who satisfy the other criteria.

Youth, relative to the average age for joint replacement, is a recognized risk factor for implant survival both in UKA and TKA [23]. Therefore it is not a good criterion for deciding between the two treatments. If, because of relative youth, the patient is likely to outlive the prosthesis, UKA may still be preferred because it is easier to revise than TKA.

In the Swedish Knee Arthroplasty Register survival data referred to above [23], most of the unicompartmental replacements were with fixed-bearing prostheses, some of which have proved susceptible to late failure from polyethylene wear, particularly in young active patients [24]. The linear wear rate of polyethylene in congruent mobile bearings is much lower than in fixed bearings [25,26], and failure from wear-through of an Oxford implant has rarely been reported.

Tabor et al. [27] reported 5- to 20-year results of 95 fixed-bearing UKAs stratified on the basis of age over or under 60 years at the time of surgery. The survival rate for all the implants was 93.7 per cent at 5 years, 89.8 per cent at 10 years, 85.9 per cent at 15 years, and 80.2 per cent at 20 years. There was no significant difference in survival between the two age groups at any interval.

Based on two long term studies [14,15], Price et al. [28] reported that the 10 year cumulative survival rate of a subset of 52 OUKAs in patients less than 60 years old was not significantly different from that of the remainder of the cohort aged 60 years or more (91 per cent; CI 12.4 and 96 per cent; CI 3.2 respectively). In this study, the 'young' patients were mainly in their fifties (mean age 56.4 years) and we have no significant data about patients aged 40 years or less.

We believe that, at least in patients over 50, age need not be a factor in choosing between OUKA and TKA. If the indications for OUKA are fulfilled, we prefer it at all ages.

Activity level

We have found no published evidence of the effect of activity (separately from youth) on the survival of UKA in general and have no prospective data. Like others, we advise our patients to avoid very vigorous use of the repaired knee, particularly in contact sports, but patients do not always do as they are told.

Pandit et al. [29] studied 50 consecutive patients aged less than 60 years (average 55 years) who had been followed for at least 2 years after OUKA (Phase 3). Their mean Tegner activity score was 4.1, significantly higher than the mean score (2.6) of a parallel group of OUKA patients aged over 60. More than 30 per cent of the younger patients participated in high-demand activities, such as skiing, tennis, and manual labour. If this sample of patients is similar, in respect of activity, to those under 60 years old in the long-term survival studies referred to above [28], vigorous use of an OUKA may not significantly threaten its survival.

Weight

Obesity has often figured as a contraindication to UKA but weight has not been one of our criteria for OUKA. Studies of retrieved meniscal bearings have revealed no association between patient weight and linear wear rate [25].

In Tabor's study [27], obese patients, defined as having a body mass index greater than 30, had *better* survival at all intervals than non-obese patients, with the difference reaching statistical significance at 20 years. (Females had significantly better survival than males at 10, 15, and 20 years, but the possible association between these two variables was not explored.)

Patellofemoral arthritis

Almost all authors have included 'patellofemoral arthritis' in the list of contraindications to unicompartmental arthroplasty and it may strike the reader as strange that we have not yet mentioned it.

In anteromedial OA, the patellofemoral compartment very commonly exhibits chondromalacia, fibrillation, and cartilage erosions that sometimes expose bone. These lesions are mainly on the medial longitudinal (or 'odd') and medial facets of the patella and the equivalent surfaces of the femoral trochlea (see Fig. 2.2(g)), but they are also seen astride the median ridge of the patella and in the groove of the trochlea. They are much less common on the lateral facets. Marginal osteophytes are often seen on the preoperative radiographs and even more commonly when the joint is open to inspection.

The presence of any of these lesions has frequently been taken to contraindicate unicompartmental replacement. However, there are some evidence-based arguments for believing that this is unnecessary.

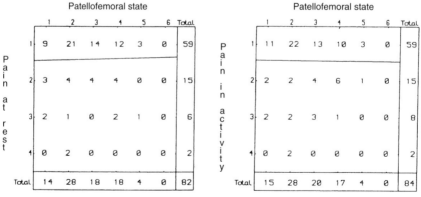

Patellofemoral state: 1 = good; 2 = moderate; 3 = poor; 4 = grossly disorganized; 5 = previous patellectomy; 6 = previously replaced.
Pain: 1 = none; 2 = mild; 3 = moderate; 4 = severe.

Figure 2.18 Patellofemoral state versus postoperative pain (a) at rest and (b) during activity. Each table is also a graph on which is plotted the linear regression line that fits the data with minimum squared error. Both lines are nearly horizontal showing that the outcome was independent of the preoperative state. (Reproduced with permission from Lippincott Williams & Wilkins from Goodfellow JW and O'Connor JJ. Clinical results of the Oxford Knee. Surface arthroplasty of the tibiofemoral joint with a meniscal bearing prosthesis. *Clin Orthop* 1986; **205**: 21–42.)

We first reached this opinion in 1986 [1] based on a study of 125 bicompartmental Oxford arthroplasties performed for OA (74) or rheumatoid arthritis (51). In these procedures only the tibiofemoral articular surfaces were replaced; the patella and the trochlea were retained. The state of the patella's articular surface was recorded intraoperatively. At postoperative review (mean follow-up 49 months) no correlation was found between the intraoperative state of the patellofemoral joint and the patients' postoperative complaints of pain (Fig. 2.18).

Despite the mixture of diagnoses in this study (and its questionable relevance to unicompartmental replacement), at that time it provided the only scientific evidence on which to base our practice. Accordingly, ever since that publication, we have continued to ignore the state of the patellofemoral joint, whether assessed radiographically or intraoperatively, when deciding between OUKA and TKA. Nor has preoperative anterior knee pain been treated as a contraindication. Despite this practice (and the similar recommendation we have given to others), patellofemoral problems have rarely been the cause of failure after OUKA.

Of the 28 revision operations reported in two series totalling 575 OUKA [14,15] none was for patellofemoral pain or malfunction. The survival tables in these two studies extended to 14 years and 17 years, respectively, and the total number of knees at risk at the tenth year was 169.

Of 50 revision operations undertaken in 699 OUKA knees, followed for up to 6 years in the Swedish Knee Arthroplasty Register, only one was for a patellofemoral problem [30].

In 28 knees, radiographs taken 1–2 years after OUKA were compared with films taken 10+ years later and no significant difference between them was found [16]. (This study was based on anteroposterior and lateral radiographs of the patellofemoral joint as 'skyline' views were not available.)

Pandit et al. [12, Chapter 6] compared fluoroscopically centred radiographs of 101 knees one year and 5 to 7 years after OUKA Phase 3 and found one case of definite progression of patellofemoral arthritis on the Altman scale and none on the Ahlback.

Discussion

Although we cannot offer a full explanation for the (apparent) enigma that the preoperative state of the patellofemoral joint has so little long-term predictive power, there are considerations that make it less inexplicable than at first sight.

First, similar lesions to those seen radiographically and intraoperatively in anteromedial OA are common in the joints of most middle-aged and elderly people and, presumably, must be compatible with adequate function. Owre [31] found flaking and fissuring of some part of the patellar cartilage at necropsy in all but one of 16 subjects aged 60–80 years. Wiles et al. [32] recorded that nearly all adult patellofemoral joints showed some pathological changes. The medial border of the medial facet was the most frequent site, and severe degeneration was associated with marginal osteophytes. Outerbridge [33] reported the state of the patellar cartilage during 101 open meniscectomies. He found 'surface fissuring and fragmentation' with increasing frequency at each decade in up to 12 of 15 subjects aged 50–69 years. Emery and Meachim [34] gave a

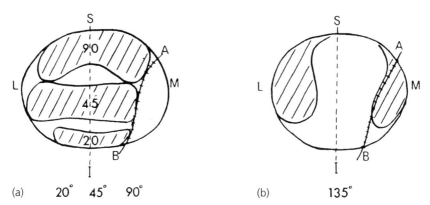

Figure 2.19 Diagrammatic representation of contact areas on the patella in varying degrees of flexion. (Reproduced with permission and copyright © of the British Editorial Society of Bone and Joint Surgery [Goodfellow JW, Hungerford DS, Zindel M. Patellofemoral joint mechanics and pathology. 1. Functional anatomy of the patellofemoral joint. *J Bone Joint Surg [Br]* 1976; **58-B**: 287–90].)

detailed description of the topography of surface degeneration at necropsy. They found fibrillation in almost every knee they examined. In young subjects degeneration was limited to the articular margins and the medial longitudinal facet of the patella, but in middle-aged subjects fibrillation was seen elsewhere on the patella surface. At these sites it became progressively more common and more severe with increasing age, frequently exposing subchondral bone. The cartilage lesions and marginal osteophytes referred to above were all chance findings at necropsy or at arthrotomy performed for reasons not associated with the patellofemoral joint. Therefore the lesions can be assumed to be generally compatible with adequate patellofemoral function. They are likely to be at least as common in the joints of candidates for unicompartmental replacement as they are in the rest of the middle-aged and elderly population, and to have as little significance.

Secondly, lesions on the medial margin of the patella may have no secondary effect on the rest of the knee joint. There are two unusual features of the medial longitudinal, or 'odd', facet. It is the *only* part of the patella's surface that articulates with the medial femoral condyle in full flexion (Fig. 2.19(b)) [35]. In anteromedial OA, the inferior surface of that condyle is devoid of cartilage, and so it is almost inevitable that the odd facet will be secondarily damaged. However, the odd facet *only* articulates with the femoral condyle, and never with the medial trochlear facet (Fig. 2.19(a)); therefore a lesion on the odd facet has no potential to cause secondary damage to the rest of the patellofemoral joint. After OUKA, the odd facet articulates in full flexion only on the metal prosthetic condyle. Therefore its circumstances are similar to those of the retained patella after TKA.

Thirdly, preoperative genu varum tends to overload the medial patellofemoral facets, the most commonly damaged surfaces [36]. Also, osteophytes at the anterior margin of the erosion on the medial femoral condyle can impinge on the medial facet of the patella in flexion. After OUKA, the varus deformity is corrected, tending to unload the medial facet, and the osteophytes are excised during the operation.

Finally, late failure of UKA caused by patellar impingement due to implant design may be wrongly attributed to progression of arthritic lesions already present at the time of surgery. In UKA models with polyradial femoral condyles, the femoral component must be mounted on the femur so that its anterior margin is flush with the retained cartilage of the trochlear facet. If this is not achieved, the patella has to negotiate a ridge as it moves distally on the femur. Hernigou and Deschamps [37] demonstrated that, if such a femoral component is implanted too far anteriorly, the patella can sustain severe damage from impingement in flexion. The technical error may only be revealed by skyline radiographs taken in 90° flexion (Fig. 2.20) and may have been overlooked in the past, with late failure from patellofemoral pain being wrongly attributed to spontaneous progression of degeneration in the patellofemoral joint. Impingement may explain the high incidence of patellofemoral deterioration reported by Berger et al. [38]. Of 49 knees treated by UKA (Miller–Galante) and followed for 10–13 years, seven (14 per cent) had radiographic evidence of progressive medial facet patellofemoral joint-space loss. Two of these knees had already been revised (at 7 and 10 years postoperatively) for anterior knee pain attributed to the patellofemoral joint. Of the remaining five, four (one lateral arthroplasty) demonstrated 'severe patellofemoral joint-space loss secondary to impinge-

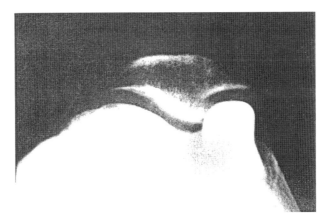

Figure 2.20 Radiograph, taken 15 years after medial arthroplasty with a polyradial fixed-bearing implant, demonstrating severe erosive changes due to impingement of the femoral component on the patella. (Reprinted with permission from The Journal of Bone and Joint Surgery, Inc [Hernigou P, Deschamps G. Patellar Impingement Following Unicompartmental Arthroplasty. *J Bone Joint Surg [Am]* 2002; **84-A**: 1132–7].)

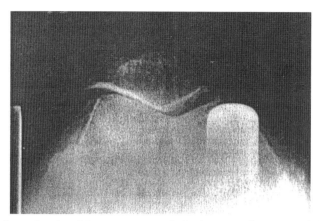

Figure 2.21 Radiograph, taken 16 years postoperatively, demonstrating osteoarthritis of the lateral part of the patellofemoral joint. Reprinted with permission from The Journal of Bone and Joint Surgery, Inc [Hernigou P, Deschamps G. Patellar Impingement Following Unicompartmental Arthroplasty. *J Bone Joint Surg [Am]* 2002; **84-A**: 1132–7].

ment with the femoral component'. These deteriorations occurred despite use of the strict preoperative selection criteria of Kozinn and Scott [39] which include '… only mild radiographic signs of deterioration of the patellofemoral joint' (Outerbridge grades 1 and 2) and absence of preoperative patellofemoral symptoms.

Unlike polyradial components, the spherical femoral component of the OUKA does not reach the medial trochlear facet of the femur (see Chapter 3, Figs. 3.6 and Appendix, A10). Therefore accurate alignment of its surface with that of the articular cartilage is not required as its anterior edge is always buried a few millimetres below the patellofemoral joint line.

Hernigou and Deschamps [37] also observed progressive OA of the patella in the second postoperative decade, quite separately from impingement. Joint-space narrowing was most commonly seen in the lateral patellofemoral compartment (Fig. 2.21). It was associated with significant symptoms, and was predicted by lack of joint congruency on the preoperative skyline radiographs. However, the symptoms from this type of degeneration were less severe than those arising from impingement and therefore no revision operation had been performed.

Conclusion

The studies referred to above support the conclusion that the presence of peripheral osteophytes, chondromalacia, fibrillation, and even full-thickness erosions in the patellofemoral compartment need not significantly prejudice the function of the knees of older people. The presence of such lesions in the joints of candidates for UKA is to be expected, and the rarity of revision of OUKA from patellofemoral symptoms, at least in the first 15 years, suggests that they can be ignored.

We now usually exclude knees in which the patellofemoral joint exhibits bone loss with eburnation and longitudinal grooving, although very few such cases have been encountered and we do not have evidence to support this practice.

Degenerative lateral meniscus

The presence of degenerative tears of the lateral meniscus has been regarded as a contraindication to UKA by some authors. Arthroscopy has not been used as a routine preoperative investigation in any published series of OUKA and, as the state of the meniscus cannot be assessed adequately through the small incision now employed, we do not have data on its predictive significance. Nevertheless, as mentioned above, the most common cause for revision of OUKA (Phase 2) was arthritis of the lateral compartment, and it is possible that a more stringent approach than we have adopted would diminish the failure rate from that cause. However, necropsy studies have shown that degenerative lesions are common in both menisci in middle-aged and older people, and so they must usually be compatible with adequate function of the joint [40]. Ritter *et al.* [41] found the lateral meniscus to be 'degenerative or absent' in 69 per cent of varus arthritic knees treated by joint replacement. Therefore paying attention to the state of the lateral meniscus would deny the advantages of UKA to very many patients in the hope of diminishing the 1.7 per cent 10-year CRR from lateral compartment failure.

We do know of instances of symptomatic meniscal tears occurring after OUKA, treated by arthroscopic meniscectomy, but we have no experience ourselves of that complication.

Chondrocalcinosis

Because chondrocalcinosis can be taken as evidence of 'inflammatory arthritis', preoperative radiographic calcification in the menisci and the articular cartilage, or calcified deposits seen at arthrotomy, have been deemed contraindications to unicompartmental replacement [42]. However, in the only study to compare the outcome of OUKA in knees with and without chondrocalcinosis [43] no difference was found.

What proportion of patients with osteoarthritic knees needing surgery is suitable for OUKA?

The proportion of osteoarthritic knees deemed suitable for medial unicompartmental arthroplasty depends on the selection criteria. Our experience, using the indications given above, is that about one-third of knees with OA severe enough to need joint replacement are suitable for OUKA. The criteria are evidence-based in that they have been employed with little variation since the 1980s and are attested by 10-year cumulative survival studies of several independent cohorts (and 15-year results in one of these) [15].

In contrast, Stern *et al.* [44] applied the often quoted criteria of Kozinn and Scott [39] to knees with OA severe enough to warrant joint replacement and found only 6 per cent suitable for UKA.

Ritter *et al.* [41] examined retrospectively the preoperative and intraoperative records of 4021 osteoarthritic varus knees treated by TKA to determine how many of them would have been 'ideal candidates' for UKA. They first applied anatomical criteria, i.e. '… a normal ACL, a normal lateral meniscus, no more than mild osteophytes in the patellofemoral and/or lateral compartment, no more than grade 2 chondromalacia in the patellofemoral compartment and no more than grade 1 chondromalacia in the lateral compartment'. Only 247 knees (6.1 per cent) met these criteria. They then applied clinical criteria attributed to Kozinn and Scott [39], i.e. patients should be more than 60 years old and weigh less than 82 kg, the flexion contracture should be less than 5°, and varus deformity less than 10°. This reduced the number to 87 knees, 2.2 per cent of the original cohort.

If, in fact, UKA were useful in as few patients as these studies suggest, few surgeons would ever see enough suitable patients to become adept in its use. However, the detailed data provided by Ritter *et al.* [41] reveal that the criteria that they applied retrospectively and those that we have used prospectively are so dissimilar that the 15-fold difference between our practice and their prediction is readily explained.

Strikingly, they found that 45 per cent of their cohort of knees had a normal ACL, the basic anatomical requirement for a successful OUKA. However, this large group was diminished to 6.1 per cent because of the presence of lateral compartment chondromalacia (74 per cent), a degenerative lateral meniscus (69 per cent), patellofemoral chondromalacia (55 per cent), lateral compartment osteophytes (33 per cent), or patellofemoral osteophytes (30 per cent), all of which can occur in middle-aged people with no knee complaints and none of which has played a part in our selection process. The clinical criteria (overweight (53 per cent), more than 5° flexion deformity (32 per cent), age (12 per cent)) that further reduced the number of suitable knees to 2.2 per cent have also all been ignored in our practice.

The contraindications criticized above were elaborated by surgeons whose experience was with fixed-bearing prostheses. Their criteria have been widely accepted and few knees outside these narrow limits may have been treated by UKA. Consequently, there is little evidence other than ours to contradict them. However, our experience has been with a meniscal-bearing prosthesis implanted (since 1987) by a fully instrumented method. The proportion of suitable cases may not be the same for fixed-bearing devices that are susceptible to medium-term polyethylene wear and patella impingement and, until recently, have been implanted with little instrumental assistance.

Other pathologies

Anteromedial OA accounts for more than 90 per cent of the knees we consider suitable for OUKA. However, there are some other pathologies for which the operation may be appropriate.

Focal spontaneous osteonecrosis of the knee

Idiopathic avascular necrosis (AVN) of the medial femoral condyle or, more rarely, of the medial tibial plateau presents anatomical features very similar to those of anteromedial OA (focal loss of bone and cartilage in the medial compartment with the ligaments intact) and therefore is theoretically suitable for OUKA (Fig. 2.22).

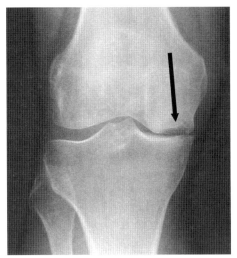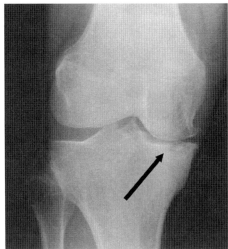

Figure 2.22 Avascular necrosis lesions in femoral and tibial condyles.

Preoperative investigation should include MRI in addition to the radiographs. Unlike anteromedial OA, varus stressed radiographs of knees with AVN lesions do not always show full-thickness cartilage loss. The MRI substantially overestimates the extent of the damage.

Marmor [45] reported generally good results in 34 knees but with four failures at a mean follow-up of 5.5 years.

Langdown et al. [46] reported the results of 29 knees with medial compartment osteonecrosis (26 femoral and three tibial) treated by OUKA (Phases 2 and 3). The mean follow-up time was 8.2 years (range 1–13 years). There had been no revisions, and the mean postoperative Oxford Knee Score (37.8 ± 7.6) was not significantly different from the score for a similar group of osteoarthritic knees (matched for age, sex, and time since surgery) also treated by OUKA (Oxford Knee Score: 0 = poor; 48 = excellent).

The surgical technique sometimes had to be modified if there was a large collapsed lesion of the femoral condyle to ensure that the first milling did not remove too much bone. We believe that large defects after curettage of dead bone are best filled with cement rather than graft using the bone removed at surgery.

Failed upper tibial osteotomy

We, and others, have used OUKA for the revision of knees with persistent symptoms after valgus osteotomy of the upper tibia, although there have been few reports on the outcome.

Thornhill and Scott [47], using the Brigham implant, referred to some successes but noted technical problems with ligamentous instability.

Vorlat et al. [48] reviewed 38 medial OUKAs of which six were performed on knees with failed high tibial osteotomy (HTO). Two of these had to be revised because of progression of arthritis in the lateral compartment. The failure rate of 33 per cent in the HTO group was compared with a 6.3 per cent failure rate in the group with primary OA.

Rees *et al.* [49] collected data (from three sources) on 631 OUKAs, 18 of which had been performed for failed HTO and the remainder for primary anteromedial OA. The reason for revision of the original HTO was persistent medial pain in every case, and in all but one there had been undercorrection of the varus deformity. The mean cumulative follow-up times of the two groups were similar (5.6 years and 5.4 years, respectively) and there were no significant differences between their mean ages or sex ratios. The mean time to revision was 2.9 years for the HTO group (five knees) and 4.1 years for the primary OA group (19 knees). The cumulative survival rates at 10 years were 66 per cent and 96 per cent, respectively (log rank comparison $P < 0.0001$). The reason for all the OUKA failures in the HTO group was persistent pain.

Accelerated lateral wear has been reported by Lynskey (personal communication), who described one OUKA, performed for failed HTO, in which the lateral compartment wore away so that the staples from the previous closing-wedge osteotomy became visible in the joint. The explanation for this mode of failure may be biomechanical. OUKA corrects the varus deformity intra-articularly. If the varus has already been corrected (even partially) by an extra-articular osteotomy, valgus alignment may result, with overloading of the lateral compartment.

We believe that previous tibial osteotomy is a contraindication to OUKA. The revision rate of 34 per cent at a mean follow-up of 5.4 years is much worse than the results reported for TKA after HTO by Meding *et al.* [50]. They reported one implant failure in 33 knees followed for a mean of 8.7 years after TKA revision of failed tibial osteotomies.

Post-traumatic osteoarthritis

Medial compartment OA following intra-articular tibial plateau fracture suggests itself as suitable for OUKA and some cases have been treated. The number is low because the medial condyle is less often fractured than the lateral condyle. Limitation of the flexion range is not uncommon after intra-articular fracture and excludes some cases, as would coincidental ligament damage.

The results have been variable, and we have too few data either to support or reject this pathology as an occasional indication.

Traumatic ruptured ACL plus secondary unicompartmental OA

ACL rupture followed by degeneration of the medial compartment is the reverse of the sequence seen in primary anteromedial OA, and the anatomy of the arthritic lesions in the two disorders is different, with the cartilage erosions being sited in the posteromedial quadrant of the knee.

We, and others, have treated a few such cases, in relatively young patients, by replacement of the ACL (with a tendon graft) and resurfacing of the medial compartment (with OUKA). The ligament replacement and the resurfacing procedure can be done at the same time or in two stages. If instability is the main symptom, it may be best to replace the ligament first and perform the arthroplasty after an interval, if pain persists, and only if knee stability has been achieved. If, as is usually the case, pain is the main problem, it is probably better to carry out the two procedures together.

The operation is attractive to relatively young patients who hope to delay (or avoid) TKA, but there are no published series on which to base the practice. Our experience is not adequate to propose this treatment or to comment on the long-term outcome.

Lateral unicompartmental osteoarthritis

Lateral unicompartmental OA is a relatively rare disease, accounting for less than 10 per cent of all unicompartmental arthritis. The clinical results of UKA in the lateral compartment have sometimes been worse than in the medial compartment [51] and sometimes better [52]. Some early papers reported results of series containing both medial and lateral operations as if they were essentially the same, but the normal anatomy and the pathological lesions of the two compartments are very different.

Normal anatomy

Whereas some fibres of the MCL are tight throughout the range of movement, all the fibres of the LCL slacken at about 20° flexion. Lacking an equivalent of the MCL, the lateral compartment depends for stability in flexion upon dynamic structures such as the iliotibial band and the popliteus muscle. As a consequence, in the absence of muscle activity, varus load can cause wide distraction of the lateral articular surfaces (Fig. 2.23).

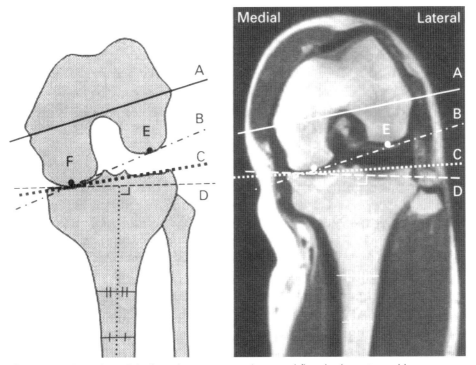

Figure 2.23 Distraction of the lateral compartment in normal flexed valgus-stressed knee. (Reproduced with permission and copyright © of the British Editorial Society of Bone and Joint Surgery [Tokuhara Y, Kadoya Y, Nakagawa S, Kobayashi S and Takaoka K. The flexion gap in normal knees. An MRI study. *J Bone Joint Surg [Br]* 2004; **86-B**: 1133–6].)

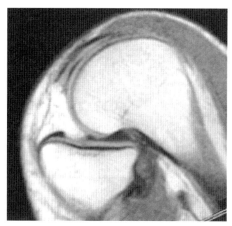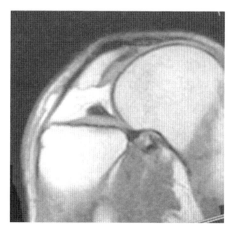

Figure 2.24 In the normal knee, the lateral condyle (right), unlike the medial condyle (left), rolls off the back of the tibial plateau in full flexion (Dr Y Kayoda, personal communication).

The medial plateau is slightly concave but the lateral plateau is convex. The lateral meniscus is more mobile than the medial meniscus, and its excursion during flexion–extension and axial rotation is greater than that of the medial meniscus. In high flexion (>120°), the lateral femoral condyle rolls over the posterior lip of the lateral plateau onto the posterior surface of the tibia (Fig. 2.24), taking the posterior horn of the meniscus with it. By contrast the posterior excursion of the medial meniscus ceases at about 90 flexion, and the medial condyle, and its meniscus, stay on the upper surface of the tibia.

Pathology

Patients are predominantly female. Flexion deformity is less common and hyperextension is sometimes seen. The valgus deformity is usually correctible manually.

The pattern of cartilage and bone erosion seen in anteromedial arthritis is not found on the lateral side [5]. Lateral unicompartmental OA is a disease of the areas of contact in flexion; the cartilage and bone erosions are in the central part of the tibial plateau, not anteriorly. The posterior surface of the femoral condyle is usually involved, and its inferior surface may be preserved.

Results

The results for 53 knees with lateral OA treated by OUKA (Phases 1 and 2) were reported in 1996 [53] with a mean follow-up of 5 years. Eleven knees had required revision, six for dislocation of the bearing, three for late infection, one for loosening of the tibial component, and one for a stress fracture. Figure 2.25 shows the most common form of dislocation of the lateral bearing. (Displacement of a medial bearing into the intercondylar space is rare.)

At 5 years, when there were 23 knees still at risk, the cumulative survival rate was 82 ± 15.4 per cent. The main reason for the poor survival was the bearing dislocation rate of 10 per cent. All the dislocations occurred in the first 12 months after operation. The knees in which no dislocation (and no infection) occurred had a cumulative survival of 98 per cent and their clinical scores were as good as those reported for the medial OUKA.

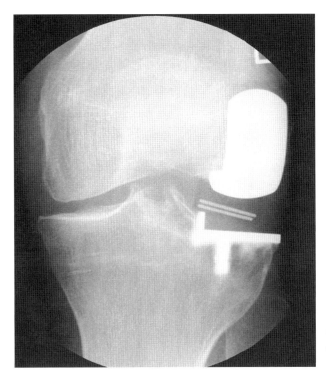

Figure 2.25 Lateral bearing dislocated into the intercondylar space.

Comment

The mobile bearing of the OUKA prosthesis depends on limited separation of the articular surfaces to keep it in place, and so it is not surprising that the bearing dislocation rate laterally was 10 times that in the medial compartment. However, it is difficult to explain why dislocation only occurred in the first year, and why those knees that survived that period did not dislocate later. Robinson *et al.* [54] reviewed the radiographs of the patients reported by Gunther *et al.* [53] and found that bearing dislocation was associated with the height of the prosthetic joint line laterally, i.e. 'The mean proximal tibial varus angle for knees the bearings of which had dislocated was 9° and for those which had not was 5°. In both groups it was greater than was expected in the normal knee'. They suggested that the technique of ligament balancing, although successful in the medial compartment, resulted in an elevated prosthetic joint line and stretching of the more compliant lateral structures.

The good results achieved in those knees in which the bearing did not dislocate were confirmed by Robinson *et al.* [55] in their study of five knees 10+ years after lateral OUKA. Video fluoroscopy showed the normal relationship throughout the range of movement between patellar tendon/tibial angle and flexion angle, typical of the normal kinematics of the knee in the sagittal plane [36] (see Fig. 1.18).

We do not, now, recommend OUKA for the treatment of lateral unicompartmental arthritis. Neither the Phase 3 tibial component nor the Phase 3 bearings are suitable for use in the lateral compartment. One alternative is to use a tibial implant with a fixed-bearing surface, avoiding dislocation at the expense of risking medium-term failure from

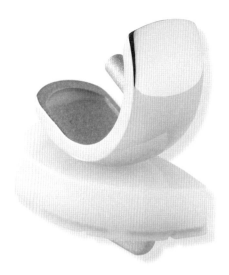

Figure 2.26 The fixed-bearing Vanguard M tibial component articulating with the OUKA femoral component.

polyethylene wear. A fixed-bearing tibial component (Fig. 2.26) is available for use with the Oxford Phase 3 femoral component, employing similar instruments and the same principles of implantation. We do not have statistical evidence to support this solution.

We have recently developed a lateral OUKA with a spherically convex tibial component and a biconcave mobile bearing. The implant is currently under assessment using modified instruments and a surgical technique that avoids the elevation of the prosthetic joint line observed by Robinson *et al.* [55].

Contraindications

In this chapter we have preferred to deal with patient selection by describing mainly the positive indications for OUKA rather than its contraindications. For completeness, the following list brings together all the contraindications, most of which have already been discussed or implied.

General

All the general contraindications recognized in the practice of joint replacement surgery apply to unicompartmental replacement and are not rehearsed exhaustively here.

Among them, OUKA (like TKA) is likely to fail in limbs with sensory and /or motor neurological impairment.

The use of a tourniquet during the operation, almost a necessity for OUKA (Phase 3) performed through a small incision, is dangerous in limbs with vascular insufficiency. It may also be dangerous to apply tourniquets to both lower limbs, and for this reason we seldom perform bilateral OUKA in one session, preferring to stage the procedures with an interval of not less than 6 weeks.

Particular

Unicompartmental arthroplasty is contraindicated in the inflammatory forms of arthritis because they are diseases of the synovium and therefore cannot be limited to one compartment. However, the loss of cartilage in early rheumatoid arthritis can be unicompartmental and has been mistaken for anteromedial OA and treated by OUKA [56]. The clinician needs to be aware of this pitfall because it results in early failure due to involvement of the other compartments of the knee.

We have already noted the anatomical contraindications listed below:

- absent or severely damaged ACL (or PCL or MCL)
- failure to demonstrate eburnated bone-on-bone contact in the medial compartment
- intra-articular varus not fully correctable
- mediolateral subluxation, not corrected on valgus-stressed films
- flexion deformity >15°
- flexion range <100° (under anaesthesia)
- thinning or erosion of central cartilage in the lateral compartment
- bone loss with eburnation and ridging in the patellofemoral joint
- previous valgus tibial osteotomy.

References

1. Goodfellow JW, O'Connor J. Clinical results of the Oxford knee. Surface arthroplasty of the tibiofemoral joint with a meniscal bearing prosthesis. *Clin Orthop* 1986; **205**: 21–42.
2. Goodfellow J, O'Connor J. The anterior cruciate ligament in knee arthroplasty. A risk-factor with unconstrained meniscal prostheses. *Clin Orthop* 1992; **276**: 245–52.
3. Goodfellow JW, Tibrewal SB, Sherman KP, O'Connor JJ. Unicompartmental Oxford Meniscal Knee arthroplasty. *J Arthroplasty* 1987; **2**: 1–9.
4. White SH, Ludkowski PF, Goodfellow JW. Anteromedial osteoarthritis of the knee. *J Bone Joint Surg [Br]* 1991; **73-B**: 582–6.
5. Harman MK, Markovich GD, Banks SA, Hodge WA. Wear patterns on tibial plateaus from varus and valgus osteoarthritic knees. *Clin Orthop* 1998; **352**: 149–58.
6. Keys GW, Carr AJ, Miller RK, Goodfellow JW. The radiographic classification of medial gonarthrosis. Correlation with operation methods in 200 knees. *Acta Orthop Scand* 1992; **63**: 497–501.
7. Deschamps G, Lapeyre B. Rupture of the anterior cruciate ligament: a frequently unrecognised cause of failure of unicompartmental knee prostheses. *Fr J Orthop Surg* 1987; **1**: 323–330.
8. Robinson D, Halperin N, Nevo Z. Devascularization of the anterior cruciate ligament by synovial stripping in rabbits. An experimental model. *Acta Orthop Scand* 1992; **63**: 502–6.
9. Gibson PH, Goodfellow JW. Stress radiography in degenerative arthritis of the knee. *J Bone Joint Surg [Br]* 1986; **68-B**: 608–9.
10. Thomas RH, Resnick D, Alazraki NP, Daniel D, Greenfield R. Compartmental evaluation of osteoarthritis of the knee. A comparative study of available diagnostic modalities. *Radiology* 1975; **116**: 585–94.
11. Dacre JE, Cushnaghan J, Jack MJ, Kirwan JR, Dieppe PA. Knee X-rays. Should we take them lying down? *Br J Rheumatol* 1991; **30** (Abstr Suppl 1): 3.

12. Jacobsen K. Gonylaxometry. Stress radiographic measurement of passive stability in the knee joints of normal subjects and patients with ligament injuries. Accuracy and range of application. *Acta Orthop Scand Suppl* 1981; **194**: 1–263.

13. Sharpe I, Tyrrell PN, White SH. Magnetic resonance imaging assessment for unicompartmental knee replacement: a limited role. *Knee* 2001; **8**: 213–18.

14. Murray DW, Goodfellow JW, O'Connor JJ. The Oxford medial unicompartmental arthroplasty: a ten-year survival study. *J Bone Joint Surg [Br]* 1998; **80-B**: 983–9.

15. Svard UC, Price AJ. Oxford medial unicompartmental knee arthroplasty. A survival analysis of an independent series. *J Bone Joint Surg [Br]* 2001; **83-B**: 191–4.

16. Weale AE, Murray DW, Crawford R, Psychoyios V, Bonomo A, Howell G, O'Connor J, Goodfellow JW. Does arthritis progress in the retained compartments after 'Oxford' medial unicompartmental arthroplasty? A clinical and radiological study with a minimum ten-year follow-up. *J Bone Joint Surg [Br]* 1999; **81-B**: 783–9.

17. Ahlback S. Osteoarthitis of the knee: a radiographic investigation. *Acta Radiol Suppl* 1968; **277**: 7–72.

18. Altman RD, Fries JF, Bloch DA, Carstens J, Cooke TD, Genant H, Gofton P, Groth H, McShane DJ, Murphy WA *et al.* Radiographic assessment of progression in osteoarthritis. *Arthritis Rheum* 1987; **30**: 1214–25.

19. Emerson RH Jr, Hansborough T, Reitman RD, Rosenfeldt W, Higgins LL. Comparison of a mobile with a fixed-bearing unicompartmental knee implant. *Clin Orthop* 2002; **404**: 62–70.

20. Kennedy WR, White RP. Unicompartmental arthroplasty of the knee. Postoperative alignment and its influence on overall results. *Clin Orthop* 1987; **221**: 278–85.

21. Hernigou P, Deschamps G. Alignment influences wear in the knee after medial unicompartmental arthroplasty. *Clin Orthop* 2004; **423**: 161–5.

22. Sisto DJ, Blazina ME, Heskiaoff D, Hirsh LC. Unicompartment arthroplasty for osteoarthrosis of the knee. *Clin Orthop* 1993; **286**: 149–53.

23. Lidgren L, Knutson K, Robertsson O. *Swedish Knee Arthroplasty Register: Annual Report 2004.* Lund: Swedish Knee Arthroplasty Register, 2004.

24. Witvoet J, Peyrache MD, Nizard R. [Single-compartment 'Lotus' type knee prosthesis in the treatment of lateralized gonarthrosis: results in 135 cases with a mean follow-up of 4.6 years]. *Rev Chir Orthop Reparatrice Appar Mot* 1993; **79**: 565–76.

25. Argenson JN, O'Connor JJ. Polyethylene wear in meniscal knee replacement. A one to nine-year retrieval analysis of the Oxford knee. *J Bone Joint Surg [Br]* 1992; **74-B**: 228–32.

26. Psychoyios V, Crawford RW, O'Connor JJ, Murray DW. Wear of congruent meniscal bearings in unicompartmental knee arthroplasty: a retrieval study of 16 specimens. *J Bone Joint Surg [Br]* 1998; **80-B**: 976–82.

27. Tabor OB Jr, Tabor OB, Bernard M, Wan JY. Unicompartmental knee arthroplasty: long-term success in middle-age and obese patients. *J Surg Orthop Adv* 2005; **14**: 59–63.

28. Price AJ, Dodd CAF, Svard UGC, Murray DW. Oxford Unicompartmental arthroplasty in patients younger than 60 years of age. *J Bone Joint Surg* [Br] 2005; **87-B**: 1488–92.

29. Pandit HG, Price AJ, Rees JL, Beard DJ, Gill HS, Dodd CAF, Murray DW. Is unicompartmental knee arthroplasty contraindicated in young active patients? *J Bone Joint Surg [Br]* 2004; **86-B** (Suppl I): 12.

30. Lewold S, Goodman S, Knutson K, Robertsson O, Lidgren L. Oxford meniscal bearing knee versus the Marmor knee in unicompartmental arthroplasty for arthrosis. A Swedish multicenter survival study. *J Arthroplasty* 1995; **10**: 722–31.

31. Owre A. Chondromalacia patellae. *Acta Chirurg Scand* 1936; **Suppl 41**.

32. Wiles P, Andrews PS, Devas MB. Chondromalacia of the patella. *J Bone Joint Surg [Br]* 1956; **38-B**: 95–113.

33. Outerbridge RE. The aetiology of chondromalacia patellae. *J Bone Joint Surg [Br]* 1961; **43-B**: 752–7.

34. Emery IH, Meachim G. Surface morphology and topography of patello-femoral cartilage fibrillation in Liverpool necropsies. *J Anat* 1973; **116**: 103–20.

35. Goodfellow J, Hungerford DS, Zindel M. Patello-femoral joint mechanics and pathology. 1: Functional anatomy of the patello-femoral joint. *J Bone Joint Surg [Br]* 1976; **58-B**: 287–90.

36. Miller RK, Goodfellow JW, Murray DW, O'Connor JJ. *In vitro* measurement of patellofemoral force after three types of knee replacement. *J Bone Joint Surg [Br]* 1998; **80-B**: 900–6.

37. Hernigou P, Deschamps G. Patellar impingement following unicompartmental arthroplasty. *J Bone Joint Surg [Am]* 2002; **84-A**: 1132–7.

38. Berger RA, Meneghini RM, Jacobs JJ, Sheinkop MB, Della Valle CJ, Rosenberg AG, Galante JO. Results of unicompartmental knee arthroplasty at a minimum of ten years of follow-up. *J Bone Joint Surg [Am]* 2005; **87-A**: 999–1006.

39. Kozinn SC, Scott R. Unicondylar knee arthroplasty. *J Bone Joint Surg [Am]* 1989; **71-A**: 145–50.

40. Noble J, Hamblen DL. The pathology of the degenerate meniscus lesion. *J Bone Joint Surg [Br]* 1975; **57-B**: 180–6.

41. Ritter MA, Faris PM, Thong AE, Davis KE, Meding JB, Berend ME. Intra-operative findings in varus osteoarthritis of the knee. An analysis of pre-operative alignment in potential candidates for unicompartmental arthroplasty. *J Bone Joint Surg [Br]* 2004; **86-B**: 43–7.

42. Kozinn SC, Marx C, Scott RD. Unicompartmental knee arthroplasty. A 4.5–6-year follow-up study with a metal-backed tibial component. *J Arthroplasty* 1989; **4**(Suppl): S1–10.

43. Woods D, Wallace D, Woods C, McLardy-Smith P, Carr AJ, Murray DW, Martin J, Gunther T. Chondrocalcinosis and medial unicompartmental knee arthroplasty. *Knee* 1995; **2**: 117–19.

44. Stern SH, Becker MW, Insall JN. Unicondylar knee arthroplasty. An evaluation of selection criteria. *Clin Orthop* 1993; **286**: 143–8.

45. Marmor L. Unicompartmental arthroplasty for osteonecrosis of the knee joint. *Clin Orthop* 1993; **294**: 247–53.

46. Langdown AJ, Pandit HG, Price AJ, Dodd CAF, Murray DW, Svard U, Gibbons CLMH. Oxford medial unicompartmental arthroplasty for focal spontaneous osteonecrosis of the knee. *Acta Orthop* 2005; **76**: 688–92.

47. Thornhill TS, Scott RD. Unicompartmental total knee arthroplasty. *Orthop Clin North Am* 1989; **20**: 245–56.

48. Vorlat P, Verdonk R, Schauvlieghe H. The Oxford unicompartmental knee prosthesis: a 5-year follow-up. *Knee Surg Sports Traumatol Arthrosc* 2000; **8**: 154–8.

49. Rees JL, Price AJ, Lynskey TG, Svard UC, Dodd CA, Murray DW. Medial unicompartmental arthroplasty after failed high tibial osteotomy. *J Bone Joint Surg [Br]* 2001; **83-B**: 1034–6.

50. Meding JB, Keating EM, Ritter MA, Faris PM. Total knee arthroplasty after high tibial osteotomy. *Clin Orthop* 2000; **375**: 175–84.

51. Scott RD, Santore RF. Unicondylar unicompartmental replacement for osteoarthritis of the knee. *J Bone Joint Surg [Am]* 1981; **63-A**: 536–44.

52. Jonsson GT. Compartmental arthroplasty for gonarthrosis. *Acta Orthop Scand Suppl* 1981; **193**: 1–110.

53. Gunther TV, Murray DM, Miller R, Wallace DA, Carr AJ, O'Connor JJ, McLardy-Smith PS, Goodfellow JW. Lateral compartment arthroplasty with the Oxford Meniscal Knee. *Knee* 1996; **3**: 33–39.

54. Robinson BJ, Rees JL, Price AJ, Beard DJ, Murray DW, McLardy-Smith P, Dodd CA. Dislocation of the bearing of the Oxford lateral unicompartmental arthroplasty. A radiological assessment. *J Bone Joint Surg [Br]* 2002; **84-B**: 653–7.

55. Robinson BJ, Rees JL, Price AJ, Beard DJ, Murray DM. A kinematic study of lateral unicompartmental arthroplasty. *Knee* 2002; **9**: 237–40.

56. Kumar A, Fiddian NJ. Medial unicompartmental arthroplasty of the knee. *Knee* 1999; **6**: 21–23.

3

3

Principles of the Oxford operation

This section is intended to be read in parallel with the description of the operative technique (Chapter 4). That chapter is concerned with 'how' to do the operation; this chapter provides the rationale—'why' the various steps of the procedure are necessary.

Although the surgeon operates exclusively on the bones, carefully avoiding any interference with the ligaments, the operation is essentially about 'soft tissue balance'. The aim is to implant the prosthetic surfaces so that the ligaments are at their resting tensions throughout the range of passive movement. This will restore both normal alignment and normal stability.

In what follows, we will often refer to the 'gap' between the medial femoral and tibial condyles, meaning the space between them created by distraction of their surfaces. With the muscles relaxed, the width of this gap can be used as a measure of the lengths of the ligaments spanning it.

The ligaments

The normal intact knee

In full extension, most of the fibres of the ligaments of the normal knee are just tight (i.e. at their resting unstretched lengths), and neither the medial nor the lateral joint surfaces can be separated. With the knee flexed (beyond about 20°) all the fibres of the posterior capsule and the LCL slacken, and distraction of the articular surfaces produces a gap (about 1 mm wide) in either compartment. These 'physiological' gaps are limited by the compliance of the other three ligaments that span the joint (the MCL and the cruciates), some of whose fibres maintain their resting tension throughout the range of flexion (see Appendix).

The effect of increasing flexion on the width of these gaps is different in the two compartments.

In the **lateral compartment,** the gap produced by distraction increases with increasing flexion to about 7 mm at 90° (mean 6.7 ± 1.9 mm) (Fig. 3.1(b)) [1].

In the **medial compartment,** the width of the gap does not alter significantly throughout the range of flexion, measuring only about 2 mm at 90° (mean 2.1 mm ±1.1 mm) (Fig. 3.1(c)).

Since the LCL and the posterior capsule are demonstrably slack in the flexed knee, the constant width of the medial gap (20°–90°) implies that the MCL and the cruciates exert a net isometric effect on that compartment throughout that range of movement. After

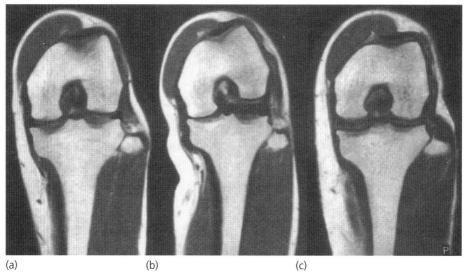

(a)   (b)   (c)

Figure 3.1 Representative MR scans in (a) a neutral position, (b) under passive varus stress, and (c) under passive valgus stress. (Reproduced with permission and copyright © of the British Editorial Society of Bone and Joint Surgery [Tokuhara Y, Kadoya Y, Nakagawa S, Kobayashi S and Takaoka K. The flexion gap in normal knees. An MRI study. *J Bone Joint Surg [Br]* 2004; **86-B**: 1133–6].)

medial unicompartmental replacement, both the stability of the knee and the entrapment of the free bearing depend upon reproducing this isometric mechanism. (The difference between the compliance of the two compartments in flexion explains why bearing dislocation is a problem laterally.)

The knee with anteromedial osteoarthritis

In anteromedial OA, the MCL and the cruciate ligaments are intact and have the same mechanical effects as in the normal joint. However, the posterior capsule is shortened. The effect of this is to close down the medial compartment gap *before full extension is reached* (Figs. 3.2(a) and 3.2(b)). For this reason, we assess the gap with the knee flexed at 20° to ensure that the posterior capsule is slack (Fig. 3.2(c)). (A flexion deformity of less than 15° is one of the criteria for OUKA, and so 20° flexion should always achieve this.)

In all positions of flexion greater than 20°, the medial condyles can be distracted the same distance as in the normal knee because the gap is limited by the normal MCL and cruciates. Therefore, distraction in flexion (Fig. 3.2(c)) restores normal alignment of the leg (Fig. 3.2(d)). The medial gap appears wider than normal only because cartilage and bone have been lost from the joint surfaces.

Balancing the ligaments in TKA and OUK

In TKA, the term 'ligament balancing' usually implies elongation of the MCL by medial release to match the length of the LCL so that, at 90° flexion, the medial and lateral gaps are equal (the flexion gap is quadrilateral). As Figure 3.3 demonstrates, this is not the physiological state.

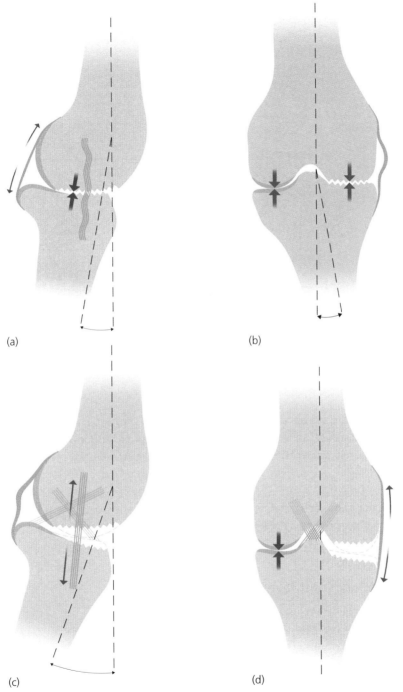

(a)

(b)

(c)

(d)

Figure 3.2 (a) With the knee extended, as far as possible, the shortened posterior capsule closes down the medial gap before full extension is reached, causing a flexion deformity, and a varus deformity that is not correctible although the MCL is slack (b). At 20 degrees flexion, however, the posterior capsule is slack (c) and an applied valgus force can distract the damage medial articular surfaces. Because the MCL is of normal length, this corrects the varus deformity (d).

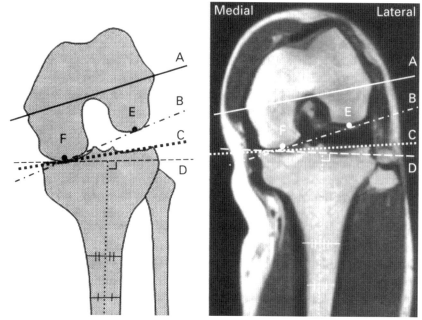

Figure 3.3 Diagram and MRI scan showing the reference lines and reference points which were used to assess the shape and width of the flexion gap. (Reproduced with permission and copyright © of the British Editorial Society of Bone and Joint Surgery [Tokuhara Y, Kadoya Y, Nakagawa S, Kobayashi S and Takaoka K. The flexion gap in normal knees. An MRI study. *J Bone Joint Surg [Br]* 2004; **86-B**: 1133–6].)

In OUKA, medial release should never be undertaken. The MCL is normal in antero-medial OA, and stability of the joint, alignment of the leg, and entrapment of the bearing all depend upon its integrity. *Balancing the ligaments means adjusting the position of the femoral component on the femur so that the medial distraction gap is the same at 20° and at 90° flexion.*

Because the lateral collateral ligament plays no part in the balancing of ligaments in OUKA, it is not represented on any of the explanatory diagrams.

The joint level

The prosthetic joint level

The prosthetic joint level is shown in the construct in Figure 3.4[1]. It is at the interface between the femoral component and the polyethylene bearing, the level at which flexion–extension occurs. The operation aims to remove enough bone from the femoral and tibial condyles to create a distraction gap, at 90° flexion, that the constructed implant will just fill. In this respect, the thickness of bone removed from the tibia is not critical. If more is removed than the minimum required, the widths of the 20° and 90° gaps are increased equally, and their 'balance' does not alter. A thicker bearing will be needed to restore stability, but this will affect neither the joint level nor, therefore, the kinematics of the replaced compartment (Fig. 3.4(c)).

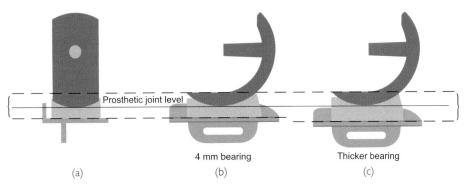

Figure 3.4 The prosthetic joint level.

The anatomical joint level

For the MCL and cruciate ligaments to resume their isometric function, the prosthesis should be implanted so that its prosthetic joint level coincides, throughout the range of movement, with the old anatomical joint level, i.e. the articular surface of the femoral condyle before it was modified by disease.

The relative thicknesses of bone removed from the posterior and the inferior surfaces of the femur is critical because it determines the relative widths of the 20° and 90° gaps.

In anteromedial OA, the posterior articular surface of the condyle is preserved (Fig. 3.5(a)). If a layer of cartilage and bone the same thickness as the metal implant is excised from the back of the condyle, the prosthetic and the anatomical joint levels will coincide (Fig. 3.5(b)). This establishes the width of the 90° gap.

The position of the anatomical joint level anteriorly is lost because all the cartilage, plus an unknown quantity of bone, has gone from the inferior surface of the femoral condyle. However, its site can be deduced because the ligaments that once matched it are still intact. As these ligaments are isometric throughout the joint range, the prosthetic joint level will be at the anatomical joint level when the gap at 20° flexion is the same as the gap (already established) at 90°. The non-articular surfaces of the femoral component are designed so that removing bone from the inferior surface of the femoral condyle widens the 20° gap without altering the 90° gap (Fig. 3.5(b)).

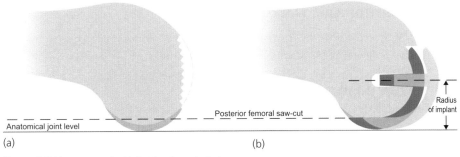

Figure 3.5 The anatomical joint level posteriorly.

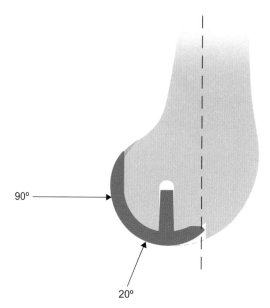

90°

20°

Figure 3.6 Effect of a spherical femoral condylar component.

Effect of using a spherical femoral component

The natural medial femoral condyle is polyradial; its inferior articular surface has a radius of curvature greater than its posterior radius. The prosthetic condyle is circular in this plane, and so the most anterior part of its articular surface cannot coincide with the old anatomical joint level but is proximal to it. Figure 3.6 shows that this does not affect the gap measurements described above, since the natural condyle is virtually circular between the points of contact at 20° and 90° (see Fig. 1.8).

The rationale of balancing the ligaments assumes that if the prosthetic and the anatomical joint levels coincide at these two points, they will also coincide at all intervening contact points, maintaining the ligaments at constant tension throughout that range. This approximation will be closest if a femoral component with a radius similar to that of the natural condyle has been chosen.

How the instruments work

We will first describe how the instruments are used to balance the ligaments, leaving aside for the moment precise orientation of the components.

The tibial saw cut

The extramedullary tibial saw guide directs a transverse saw cut below the deepest part of the anteromedial erosion. The fragment is removed and a tibial template (the same thickness as the tibial component) is laid on the cut surface (Fig. 3.7(b)). If, with the knee at

90°, a 4-mm feeler gauge can easily be inserted between the condyle and the template, sufficient tibial bone has been removed to accommodate a 4-mm bearing. (This measurement is reliable because the posterior surface of the medial femoral condyle is not eroded in anteromedial OA.)

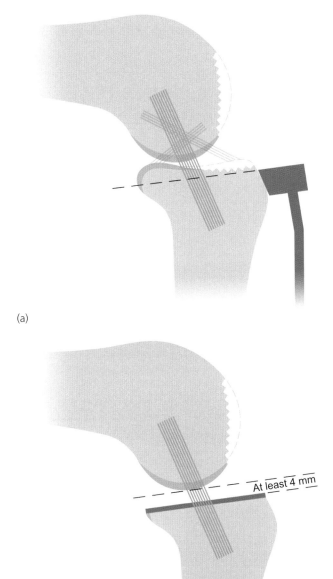

(a)

(b)

Figure 3.7 Level of tibial saw-cut.

The femoral drill guide (Fig. 3.8(a))[2]

With the knee flexed to 90°, the drill guide is applied with the upper surface of its foot touching the intact cartilage on the posterior surface of the medial femoral condyle and its face touching the eburnated bone on the inferior surface of the condyle (Fig. 3.8(a)). A drill (with a fixed collar) passes through the guide to make a hole in the bone. The axis of the hole is the same distance from the foot of the instrument as the radius of the chosen femoral component, and the depth of the hole is the same as the length of the shafts of the spigots (see below).

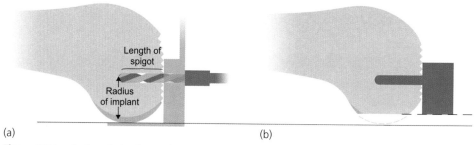

(a)   (b)

Figure 3.8 Level of posterior femoral saw-cut.

Femoral saw guide (Fig. 3.8(b))[2]

The guide is positioned in the drill hole (Fig. 3.8(b)) and directs the saw to remove from the femoral condyle a slice of bone and cartilage the same thickness as the metal of the posterior part of the femoral implant.

The concave spherical mill (Fig. 3.9)[2]

The mill is used to remove bone incrementally from the inferior surface of the femoral condyle, simultaneously shaping the bone to match the inner surface of the femoral implant. The mill rotates about a spigot inserted into the drill hole already made in the condyle.

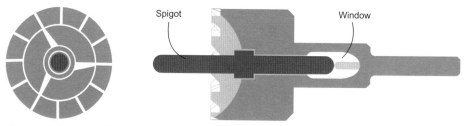

Figure 3.9 Concave spherical mill. Milling is complete when the shaft of the spigot is seen, through the window, to touch the stop.

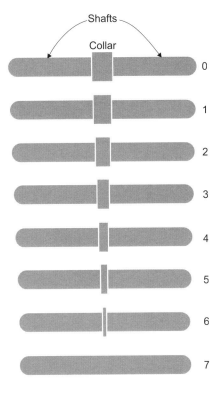

Shafts

Collar

0

1

2

3

4

5

6

7

Figure 3.10 Spigots.

The spigots (Fig. 3.10) are in a range numbered 0 to 7 depending on the thickness of the collar that acts as a stop to the mill. As the thickness of the collar decreases from 0 to 7, in 1-mm steps, the amount of bone removed increases similarly.

The lengths of both shafts of the spigots are the same, and are constant throughout the range, so they can be used either way around. The depth of the drill hole in the condyle is the same as the length of the shafts (see Fig. 3.8(a)), and so the spigots register at two sites, the surface of the condyle and the bottom of the drill hole (Fig. 3.11(a)).

The 0 spigot (the one with the thickest collar) is always used first (Fig. 3.11(b)). The mill then shapes the surface of the bone (Fig. 3.11(c)) so that a trial femoral component can be inserted (Fig. 3.11(d)). This establishes (as the spigot's number suggests) a zero point from which subsequent measurements are made. Because the contour of the arthritic condyle has been flattened by loss of bone and cartilage, the bone removed is peripheral and mostly anterior; no bone is removed centrally (Figs. 3.11(b) and 3.11(c)). After milling with the zero spigot, the articular surface of the trial femoral component lies about 5 mm distal to the eburnated surface of the bone (Fig. 3.11(d)) so that the 20° gap is smaller than the 90° gap, an essential requirement for the next step.

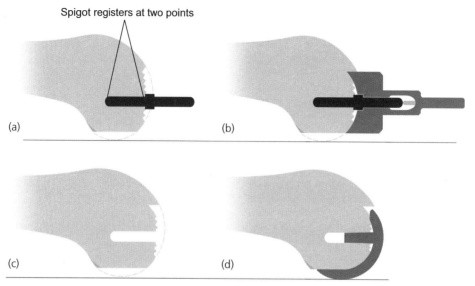

Figure 3.11 First milling.

First gap measurement (Fig. 3.12)

With both trial components in place (Fig. 3.12(a)), the 90° gap is measured (say, 5 mm). The joint is then extended and the 20° gap is measured (say, 2 mm). The difference between the 90° flexion gap and the 20° flexion gap (5 mm – 2 mm = 3 mm) gives the thickness of bone to be milled from the inferior surface of the femur to make the gaps equal. The 3 spigot (with a collar 3 mm thinner than the 0 spigot) is inserted into the drill hole and the second milling is completed (Figs. 3.12(b) and 3.12(c)).

Second gap measurement

The trial components are reinserted and the gaps are again measured; they are usually found to be the same (Fig. 3.12(d)).

Occasionally, the second measurement shows that the gap remains narrower at 20° than at 90°, and that more bone must be milled away to achieve balance. To remove a further 1 mm, the 4 spigot (with a collar 1 mm thinner than the 3 spigot) is inserted and a third milling is performed. As Figure 3.12(c) shows, the small ring of bone under the collar of the spigot escapes the second milling and has to be removed to allow the femoral component to seat. This robs the spigot of one of its points of reference. However, if a third milling has to be undertaken, the spigots continue to function as before by registering off the bottom of the drill hole. Figure 3.13 shows that, in this case, the temptation to hammer the spigot into the hole until the collar touches the bone must be resisted.

Positioning the prosthetic components

The instruments are not only designed to balance the ligaments but are also used to position each of the components precisely and predictably. These features were ignored in the above description so as to concentrate on the fundamental requirement of ligament balance.

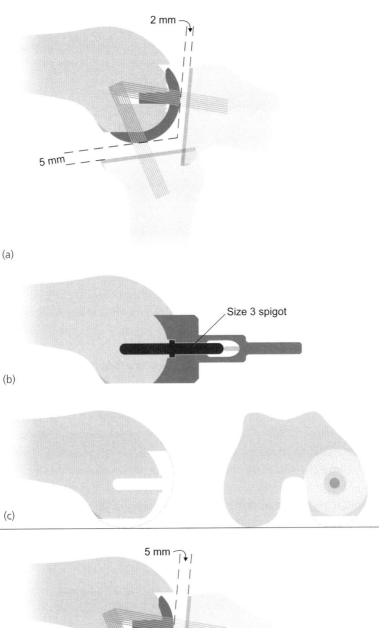

(a)

(b)

Size 3 spigot

(c)

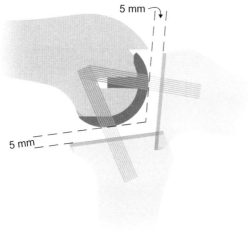

(d)

Figure 3.12 (a) First gap measurement; (b), second milling; (c) resultant bone shape; (d) second gap measurement.

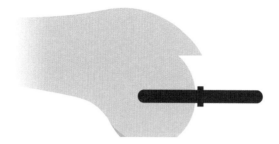

Figure 3.13 Third milling.

The tibial component

The level of the transverse tibial saw cut

In order to make space for a bearing 4 mm thick and a tibial plateau 3 mm thick, the tibial saw cut should be made about 7 mm below the original tibial articular surface[1]. However, in anteromedial OA, cartilage and bone are lost from the anterior (visible) surface of the plateau, and so the level of the saw cut cannot be measured from it. Therefore an estimate of the appropriate height is made by sawing 2–3 mm below the deepest part of the anteromedial erosion (which is readily visible to the surgeon). This gives a conservative excision which is either the right thickness or too thin.

With the knee flexed to 90° and the tibial template in place, the resulting flexion gap is measured with feeler gauges (Fig. 3.7(b)). If a 4-mm gauge cannot be inserted more bone is resected, as follows. The saw guide was fixed to the bone for the first cut with two nails driven through the lower pair of holes in the head of the guide (Fig. 3.14). To remove more bone, the guide is removed and replaced with the same pins now passing through the upper pair of holes. This displaces the guide 3 mm distally. If, after the first cut, the gap measured 1 mm, 2 mm, or 3 mm, the second cut will provide a gap suitable for a 4-mm, 5-mm, or 6-mm bearing, respectively, all of which are acceptable outcomes.

Theoretically (in a knee with anteromedial OA), the thickness of bone to be removed can be measured from the intact cartilage surface at the back of the tibial plateau. Figure 3.15 shows how a stylus attached to the tibial saw guide can be used to place the

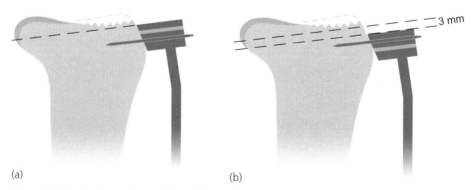

(a)   (b)

Figure 3.14 Adjusting the level of the tibial saw-cut.

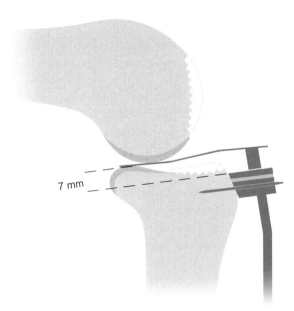

7 mm

Figure 3.15 Use of a stylus.

guide at the appropriate level. However, the posterior surface of the plateau is not visible to the surgeon and the instrument has to be positioned by feel on the intact anterior cartilage, not the meniscus. Also, the long distance from the tip of the stylus at the back of the joint to its attachment to the saw guide may cause inaccuracy because of bending.

Varus–valgus inclination

In the frontal plane, the extramedullary tibial guide aims to place the tibial plateau at about 90° to the tibial axis. In UKA, however, the alignment of the limb (tibiofemoral angle) is independent of the alignment of the plateau, and minor angular inaccuracies do not have the same significance as in TKA. The ball-and-socket configuration of the femoromeniscal articulation of the OUKA accommodates angulation of the plateau relative to the femoral component without loss of congruence (see Fig. 3.21 below).

Postero-inferior inclination

The natural medial tibial plateau is inclined backwards and downwards in the sagittal plane at a mean angle of 7°, but with a wide range of 0°–15°. In extension, the anterior position of the femoral condyle on the plateau (up the inclined plane) tends to tighten the ligaments and diminish the gap. In flexion, the posterior position of the condyle tends to slacken the ligaments. The wide range of angles recorded in the normal population might suggest that the angle of the tibial component should be 'customized' to the individual patient, to match the predisease plateau angle. However, we have always implanted the tibial plateau at the mean inclination, irrespective of the knee's anatomy, and a 7° angle is built into the tibial saw guide. As the 20° and 90° gaps are measured with the tibial template in place, the effects of this approximation on ligament tension are automatically taken into account when the gaps are balanced.

Mediolateral position (Fig. 3.16)

The mediolateral position of the tibial plateau is of importance because it determines the mediolateral position of the other two components (see below). The position is defined by the vertical saw cut (X–X in Fig. 3.16(a)). With the knee flexed at 90°, the cut is made into the intercondylar eminence, just medial to the footprint of the ACL, with the saw blade (1) touching the lateral margin of the medial femoral condyle and (2) directed towards the head of the femur. In plan view (Fig. 3.16(b)) the direction of the cut will then be in the flexion–extension plane of the knee, the approximate direction of the anteroposterior movements of the mobile bearing.

Choice of plateau size The tibial component should cover as much of the cut surface as possible to maximize the area available for the transmission of load.

It *must* reach as far as the medial cortex; therefore the implant is chosen from the range of sizes by its *width*. The plateau can overhang medially by as much as 2 mm without risk of soft tissue irritation. (More overhang than this is unnecessary as the next smaller size will fit exactly.) Some overhang is preferable to incomplete coverage.

The component *must* be placed as far back as possible so that it reaches to the posterior cortex. Full coverage is needed at this site because the bearing slides to, and beyond, the posterior edge of the plateau in flexion. In addition, very high loads may be transmitted across the flexed knee, and so the posterior part of the tibial implant needs to be supported by the posterior cortex.

The parametric range of sizes cannot always provide a component that satisfies these two criteria *and* reaches to the anterior cortex, so that often a small area of the cut surface is uncovered anterolaterally (Fig. 3.16(b)). This is not important as the bearing does not slide beyond this margin of the implant.

The bearing

The mobile bearing passively follows the track of the femoral condyle as it moves anteroposteriorly and mediolaterally relative to the plateau. The limits of these movements are set by the lengths of the ligaments, and within these limits the freedom of the bearing to translate in all directions should be unrestricted. If the bearing is unrestrained, loads are transmitted across the joint as a combination of compressive force (normal to the articular surface) and tensile forces in the soft tissues. Shear stresses at the bone–implant interfaces are thereby minimized. If bearing movement is resisted (by impingement against bone, cement, or the lateral wall of the tibial component), shear stresses develop at the femoral and/or tibial interfaces and may cause loosening of the fixed components, dislocation of the bearing and perhaps pain.

The largest translational movements of the femoral condyle are in the anteroposterior directions. The flat tibial plateau, having no anterior or posterior rim, offers

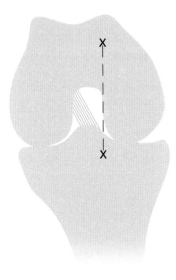

(a)

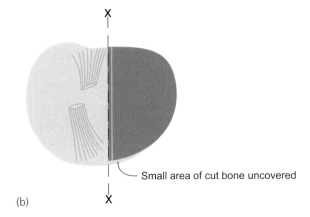

Small area of cut bone uncovered

(b)

Figure 3.16 (a) Vertical tibial saw-cut; (b) sizing and positioning the tibial component.

no limits to movement of the bearing in these directions, nor do the soft tissues interfere. In flexion, when the bearing moves posteriorly, the posterior capsule is relaxed; in extension, when the bearing moves forward, so does the anterior capsule. In a normally functioning OUKA, the excursion of the bearing regularly brings its posterior margin beyond the posterior edge of the tibial plateau in flexion, and anteromedial overhang is common in full extension (Fig. 3.17). Figure 3.17 shows that, despite these movements of the bearing, the centre of pressure always lies within the middle third of the tibial implant, maintaining the bone/implant interface in compression.

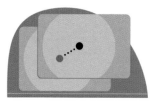

Figure 3.17 Track of bearing during flexion–extension. (The medial displacement is not to scale.)

In a knee with normally tensioned ligaments, the femoral condyle has very little freedom to translate mediolaterally, and the bearing needs equivalently little freedom to follow it. However, the forward and backward track of the bearing on the plateau during flexion–extension is not strictly anteroposterior but is inclined forwards and slightly medially (Fig. 3.17).

Rotation and entrapment

As well as the translational movements described above, the femoral condyle rotates axially relative to the tibial plateau. Obligatory internal rotation of the femur, of about 20°, occurs during extension, and a range of forced internal/external rotation is available in all flexed positions, increasing to between 20° and 30° at 90° flexion. Axial rotation of the femur relative to the tibia is accomplished by means of spinning movements at the femoromeniscal interface and anteroposterior translational movements at the meniscotibial interface. Since the femoromeniscal interface of the prosthesis is a ball-in-socket and the meniscotibial interface is flat-on-flat, spinning movements can occur at both surfaces of the bearing. One of these levels of rotation is superfluous, and so spin can be suppressed at one interface without limiting the joint's freedom to rotate. The design takes advantage of this to maximize entrapment of the bearing.

The prototype bearing (ca 1976) was circular in plan and the amount of entrapment, i.e. the height of the socket wall above its deepest point, was the same all round (Fig. 3.18(a)). However, dislocation proved more likely to occur anteriorly or posteriorly than sideways, and it was desirable to have more entrapment at the front and the back of the socket than at the sides. Furthermore, with the circular design, entrapment can only be increased by increasing the radius of the circle, and this made the bearing too large for the width of the tibial plateau. The solution was to make the bearing quadrilateral in plan, with its longer axis in the anteroposterior direction (Fig. 3.18(b)). This allowed the anterior and posterior lips of the socket to be higher (increasing anteroposterior entrapment without affecting mediolateral entrapment).

Since it is difficult to stretch the ligaments more than 2–3 mm, the posterior wall of the socket cannot provide greater entrapment than that (or the bearing cannot be inserted). Therefore the centre of the socket was moved towards the back of the quadrilateral, diminishing the height of the posterior lip and raising the anterior lip (Fig. 3.18(c)). This is the general form that the medial bearing has had ever since the Phase 1 implant was introduced in 1978.

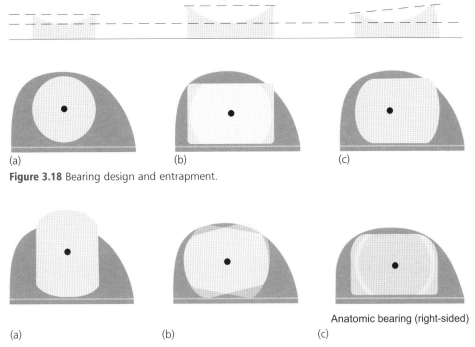

Figure 3.18 Bearing design and entrapment.

(a)   (b)   (c)

Anatomic bearing (right-sided)

(a)   (b)   (c)

Figure 3.19 Limiting rotation of the bearing.

Obviously, this mechanism can only work if the bearing maintains its anteroposterior alignment. If it spins through 90°, the socket will present reduced resistance to anterior or posterior dislocation (Fig. 3.19(a)). Figure 3.19(b) shows how its quadrilateral shape limits spin of the bearing if the centre of the socket (about which spin occurs) is close enough to the lateral wall of the tibial implant. This is achieved by positioning the femoral component appropriately. Unlimited spin is still allowed at the meniscofemoral interface and the fundamental requirement, that the bearing be free to translate in all directions, is still satisfied.

In order to minimize further the risk of bearing rotation, 'anatomic' bearings (right- and left-sided) have been introduced with an extended lateral edge (Fig. 3.19(c)). The anteromedial corner has been rounded off to minimize bearing overhang in extension and the potential for soft tissue irritation.

The femoral component

Mediolateral position

The mediolateral position of the femoral component controls the mediolateral position of the bearing on the tibial plateau. Figure 3.20 shows how the femoral drill guide ensures the correct relationship between the two fixed components.

With the knee flexed to 90° and the tibial template in place on the cut tibial plateau, the drill guide is placed so that the upper surface of its foot touches the intact

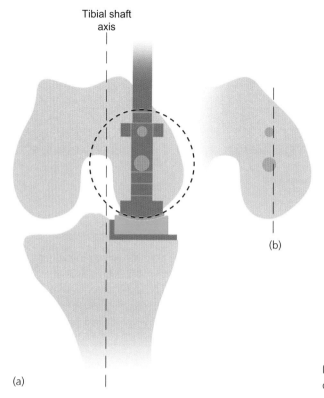

Tibial shaft
axis

(a)

(b)

Figure 3.20 Use of the femoral drill-guide.

cartilage on the posterior part of the femoral condyle (Fig. 3.8(a)). A feeler gauge (of appropriate thickness to tension the ligaments) is inserted, with its lateral surface lying against the wall of the tibial template. The convex cylindrical lower surface of the foot of the drill guide sits in the concave cylindrical upper surface of the feeler gauge, ensuring that the drill hole passes along the axis of these cylinders.

The feeler gauges are 2 mm wider than the meniscal bearings; therefore the holes drilled into the condyle locate the femoral component so that (at 90°) the bearing will lie 1 mm away from the lateral wall of the tibial component. Since extension of the knee results in a further 1–2 mm of medial translation of the bearing (see Fig. 3.17), it will always be away from the wall, but never far enough to allow it to rotate through more than 20°–30°.

Note that the mediolateral position of the femoral component must relate *precisely* to the position of the tibial component, not to the centre line of the natural femoral condyle. If the tibial component has been correctly sited, the centre of the femoral component (as represented by the larger femoral drill hole) will be *near* the centre line of the femoral condyle but not necessarily on that line (Fig. 3.20(b)).

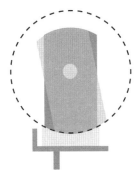

Figure 3.21 Femoral component attitude: rotation about the axis of its peg (knee flexed 90°). We consider angular alignment up to 10° acceptable.

Rotation and 'attitude'

The articular surface of the femoral component is a portion of a sphere (with its centre at the tip of its peg). The position of a spherical surface does not alter when it rotates around its centre and so, in some sense, the rotational alignment of the femoral implant is an irrelevance. Figure 3.21 shows, for instance, that rotational alignment of the femoral component about the axis of its peg does not alter the position of the bearing in the flexed knee. Nevertheless, because the femoral component is an incomplete sphere, its 'attitude' is altered by rotation in any of the three planes. The attitude of the component affects (1) the availability of its limited articular surfaces and (2) its appearance on radiographs. In two of these planes, the attitude of the component is controlled by the alignment of the femoral drill hole, into which its peg fits.

In the sagittal plane, the 'flexion–extension' attitude is correct when the peg is parallel to the long axis of the femur (Fig. 3.22). If the component is 'flexed' relative to the femoral shaft, there will be inadequate articular surface anteriorly in full extension. Conversely, if it is 'extended', there will be inadequate articular surface posteriorly for full flexion.

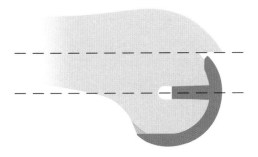

Figure 3.22 Femoral component attitude: flexion–extension.

In the frontal plane, the 'varus–valgus' attitude is correct when the peg is parallel to the mechanical axis of the femur, i.e. at approximately 7° to the long axis of the femoral shaft (Fig. 3.23). In the extended limb, this places the peg at right angles to the horizontally placed tibial component, maximizing the contact area at the meniscofemoral interface. Deviation results in diminished femoromeniscal contact area.

In the transverse plane, the axis of the peg lies in the axis of rotation and so cannot control it. The attitude of the implant, relative to the femur, is determined by the plane of the posterior femoral saw cut. The effect of rotation in producing the characteristic 'bucket-seat' appearance of the component on anteroposterior radiographs of the extended knee is discussed in Chapter 5.

All these rotations are controlled by the femoral drill guide: in the sagittal plane, by aligning the drill hole with the intramedullary rod (Fig. 3.22); in the frontal plane, by

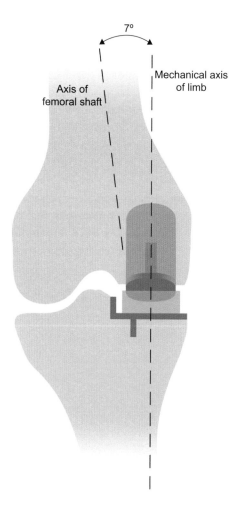

Figure 3.23 Femoral component attitude: varus-valgus.

aligning the drill hole at 7° to the intramedullary rod (Fig. 3.23); and in the transverse plane, by aligning the handle of the guide parallel to the axis of the shaft of the tibia (Fig. 3.20).

Notes

1. The thickness of the posterior facet of the femoral component varies with its radius from 5.96 mm (small) to 7.45 mm (extra large). The thickness of the tibial component (3 mm) is constant throughout the range of sizes. The thinnest bearing usually considered safe to use (4 mm) has 4.5 mm of polyethelene at its thinnest point.

2. The femoral drill guide, femoral saw guide, and concave spherical mill are all available in five sizes to match the diameters of the five sizes of femoral component.

Reference

1. Tokuhara Y, Kadoya Y, Nakagawa S, Kobayashi A, Takaoka K. The flexion gap in normal knees. An MRI study. *J Bone Joint Surg [Br]* 2004; **86-B**: 1133–6.

4

Surgical technique

Preoperative planning

The trays containing the tibial instruments and trial components are used with all sizes of femur (Fig. 4.1).

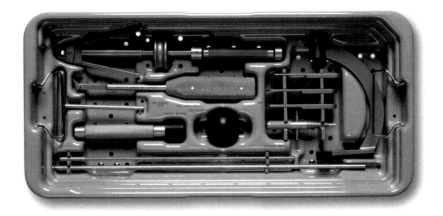

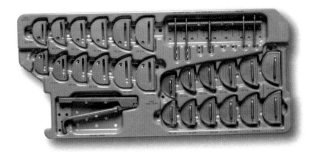

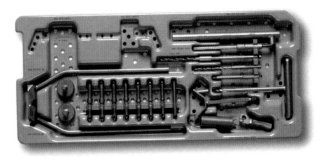

Figure 4.1

The five sizes of femoral component have different radii of curvature. For each femoral size there is a matching set of meniscal bearings in seven thicknesses, from 3 mm to 9 mm. There is a separate tray of instruments for each femoral size. The trays, three of which are shown in Fig. 4.2, contain colour coded instruments and trial components specifically for use with one size of femoral component.

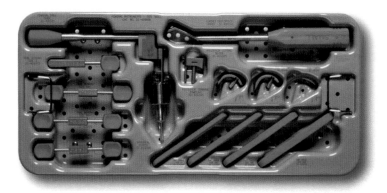

Femoral size small

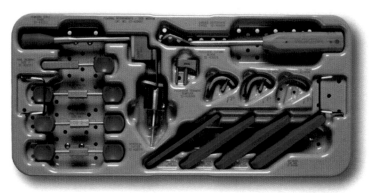

Femoral size medium

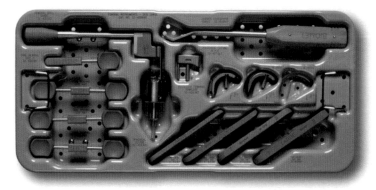

Femoral size large

Figure 4.2

X-ray template

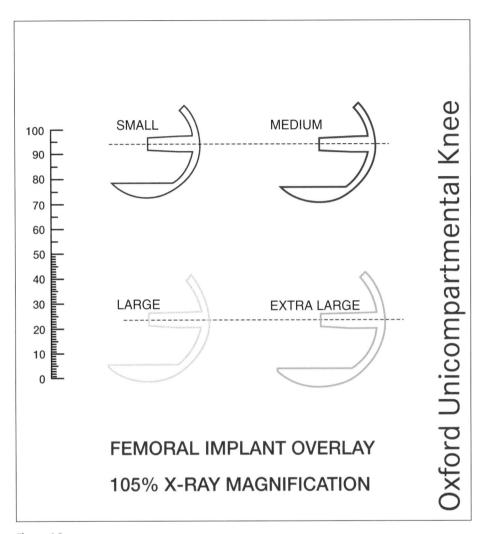

Figure 4.3

The size of femoral component should be chosen preoperatively using the X-ray template (Fig. 4.3). A true lateral radiograph is required. It should be made with the film cassette touching the lateral side of the knee and the X-ray source 100 cm from the medial side of the knee. This gives a magnification of approximately 5 per cent. If films are taken in this way, the template marked "105%" should be used. Digital images should be printed at 100 per cent for templating.

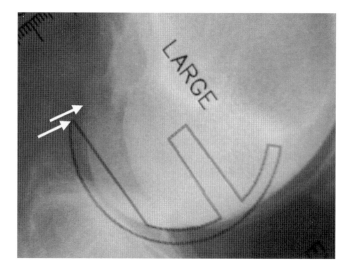

Figure 4.4

The outlines on the template are applied to the X-ray image of the medial femoral condyle. The line along the central peg of the implant should be parallel to the long axis of the femoral shaft. The outer surface of the diagrammatic component should lie about 3 mm outside the radiographic bone image, both distally and posteriorly, to allow for the thickness of articular cartilage (Fig 4.4). The ideal component is one that overhangs the bone posteriorly so it will be flush with the remaining articular cartilage.

A medium-size femoral component is appropriate for most patients. (It was, in fact, the only size used in the Phase 1 and 2 implants.)

However, in small women, it is better to employ the small size and, in large men, the large size. The extra-large and extra-small sizes are rarely used. If there is doubt between small/medium, or large/medium it is usually safer to use the medium. Similarly, if there is doubt between the extra-small and the small, or between the extra-large and the large, use the small or the large.

The operation

Positioning the limb

A thigh tourniquet is applied and the leg is placed on a thigh support with the hip flexed to about 30° and abducted, and the leg dependent. The knee must be free to flex to at least 135° (Fig. 4.5). The thigh support must not intrude into the popliteal fossa.

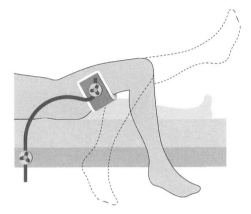

Figure 4.5

Incision

With the knee flexed to 90°, a paramedial skin incision is made from the medial margin of the patella to a point 3 cm distal to the joint line just medial to the tibial tubercle (Fig. 4.6). The incision is deepened through the joint capsule. At its upper end, the capsular incision is extended proximally for 1 to 2 cm into the vastus medialis.

Part of the retropatellar fat pad is excised and the anterior tibia is exposed. Self-retaining retractors are inserted into the synovial cavity.

The ACL can now be inspected to ascertain that it is intact. (Absence of a functioning ACL is a contraindication and the operation should be abandoned in favour of a total knee replacement.)

Large patellar osteophytes should be removed to improve access.

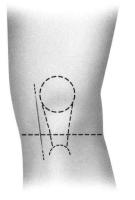

Figure 4.6

Excision of osteophytes

Large osteophytes must be removed from the
medial margin of the medial femoral condyle
and from both margins of the intercondylar notch
(Fig. 4.7). The assistant extends and flexes the knee,
moving the incision up and down, so that the
various osteophytes come into view.

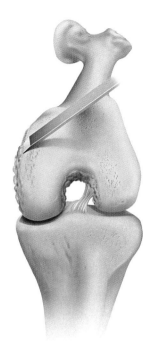

Figure 4.7

A narrow chisel (6 mm) is needed to remove the
osteophytes from beneath the medial collateral ligament (Fig. 4.8) and from the posterolateral margin of the medial condyle (to make room to insert
the saw blade into the intercondylar notch at the
next step). When removing osteophytes from
the posterolateral margin of the medial condyle
the chisel should be directed towards the femoral
head.

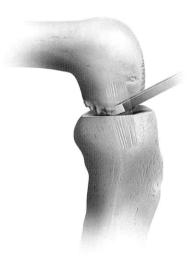

Figure 4.8

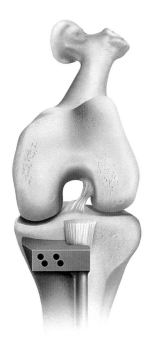

Figure 4.9

Tibial plateau resection

The front of the tibia is exposed in the lower part of the wound from the tibial tubercle to the rim of the plateau. Large osteophytes are removed from the anterior tibia as they interfere with seating of the tibial saw guide. As much as possible of the medial meniscus is excised. Do not 'release' any of the fibres of the MCL.

The tibial saw guide is applied with its shaft parallel to the long axis of the tibia in both planes (Figs. 4.9 and 4.10). (This will make the horizontal tibial saw cut slope backwards and downwards 7°.) The guide should remain in the sagittal (flexion) plane when the knee is flexed and extended.

The upper end of the guide is manipulated so that its face lies against the exposed bone. It should be pushed laterally so that the recess accommodates the patellar tendon laterally (Fig. 4.9) and, in a thin patient, the skin.

The level of resection is estimated and varies with the depth of the tibial erosion. The saw cut should pass 2 or 3 mm below the deepest part of the erosion (Fig. 4.12 and 4.14). It is better to be conservative with the first cut as the tibia can easily be re-cut if too little bone has been removed. Once the level has been decided, the guide is fixed to the bone with nails passed through the lower set of holes in its head. One nail should have a head and the other should not.

(A stylus is now available which references off intact posterior cartilage.)

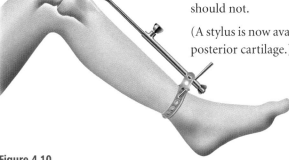

Figure 4.10

A reciprocating saw with a stiff narrow blade is used to make the vertical tibial saw cut. The blade is pushed into the intercondylar notch and must lie against the lateral margin of the medial femoral condyle (from which the osteophytes were removed). The saw cut should be medial to the origin of the ACL, avoiding damage to its fibres. The blade is pointed towards the head of the femur (Fig. 4.11), the position of which is demonstrated by the assistant who palpates halfway between the pubic tubercle and the anterior superior iliac spine.

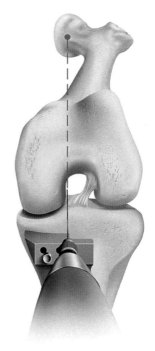

Figure 4.11

The saw must reach to the back of the tibial plateau and a little beyond. The saw cuts vertically down until it rests on the upper surface of the saw guide (Fig. 4.12). The handle of the saw must not be raised, as too deep a cut posteriorly will weaken the posterior cortex.

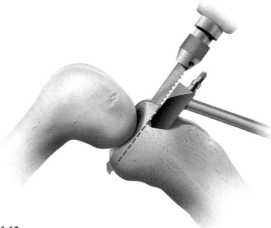

Figure 4.12

Before making the horizontal cut, a retractor is inserted between the tibia and the MCL to protect the deep fibres of the ligament from damage (Fig. 4.13).

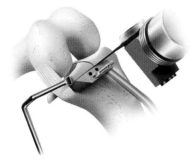

Figure 4.13

A 12-mm wide oscillating saw blade[1] is used to excise the plateau. Ensure that the blade goes right to the back of the joint. When the plateau is loose it is levered up with a broad osteotome and removed. Soft tissue attachments posteriorly may need to be cut with a knife. The posterior horn of the medial meniscus can now be removed.

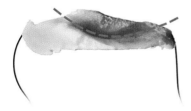

Figure 4.14

The excised plateau will show the typical lesion of anteromedial OA: eroded cartilage and bone in its middle and anterior parts and preserved cartilage posteriorly (Fig. 4.14). Osteophytes around the edge of the plateau remain attached to it when it is removed.

The excised plateau is used, with the tibial templates, to choose the size of the tibial implant by laying templates of the opposite side on its cut surface. The ideal size is one that has the correct *width*.

The thickness of bone removed from the tibia must be enough to accommodate the tibial template and a bearing at least 4 mm thick. (In a very small patient it is acceptable to use a 3-mm bearing.) To check that sufficient bone has been excised, insert the tibial template and a 4-mm feeler gauge (Fig. 4.15). (Note that whenever a feeler gauge is used to measure a gap, the retractors are removed. If they are left in, they have the effect of tightening the soft tissues which artificially diminishes the gap.)

If the 4-mm gauge cannot be inserted, or feels tight, then more bone needs to be excised from the tibia.

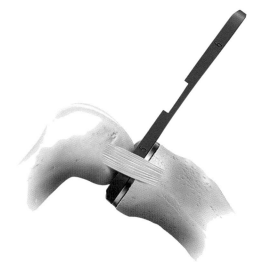

Figure 4.15

To excise more bone, the headed nail and the tibial saw guide are removed. The guide is then replaced, with the headless nail passing through one of the upper holes. The headed nail is replaced adjacent to it (in its original bone hole). This displaces the saw guide 3 mm distally (Fig. 4.16). A further layer of bone is removed and the gap is rechecked, with the tibial template in place, to ensure that at least the 4-mm feeler gauge can now be easily inserted.

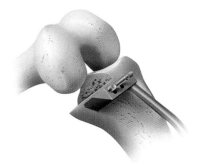

Figure 4.16

The femoral drill holes

With the knee in about 45° flexion, a hole is made into the intramedullary canal of the femur with the 5-mm awl (Fig. 4.17).

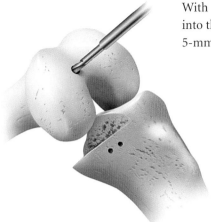

Figure 4.17

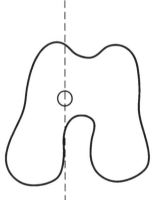
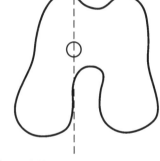

The hole must be situated 1 cm anterior to the anteromedial corner of the intercondylar notch (Fig. 4.18).

Figure 4.18

Insert the intramedullary rod until the rod pusher is stopped against the bone (Fig. 4.19).

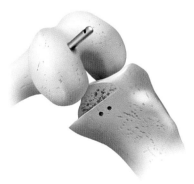

The knee is then flexed to 90°. This must be done with care as the medial border of the patella abuts against the rod which now acts as a retractor.

Figure 4.19

Replace the tibial template, insert the femoral drill guide and place a feeler gauge, 1 mm thinner than the flexion gap, between them (Fig. 4.20). **The feeler gauge must be touching the vertical wall of the tibial template**.

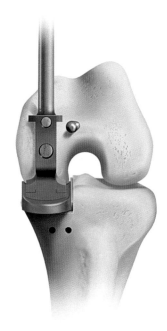

The centre of the 6-mm drill hole should lie near the centre line of the femoral condyle (i.e. in its central third), but not necessarily on the centre line. If it is not in the middle third, the position of the instruments should be checked. Occasionally osteophytes or cartilage on the posterior part of the condyle push the feeler gauge medially; they can be removed with a chisel. If the construct is too tight, a thinner feeler gauge can be used. Rarely the site of the vertical tibial saw cut should be revised.

Figure 4.20

The handle of the femoral drill guide should be aligned parallel to the long axis of the tibia (Fig. 4.20) and its **anterior face must touch the femoral condyle** (Fig. 4.21).

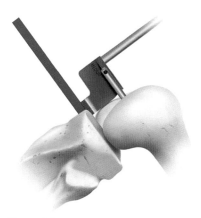

By adjusting the degree of flexion of the knee, the **upper surface of the drill guide is made to lie parallel to the intramedullary rod** when viewed from the side (Fig. 4.21).

Figure 4.21

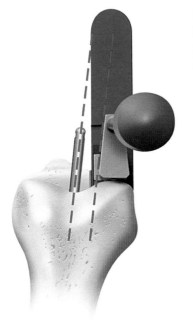

By internally and externally rotating the tibia, the **lateral surface of the 7° fin on the side of the drill guide is made to lie parallel to the intramedullary rod** when viewed from above (Fig. 4.22).

Figure 4.22

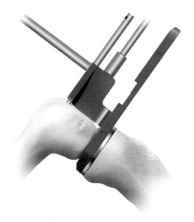

When all these six requirements are fulfilled, the 4-mm drill is passed through the upper hole in the guide, drilled into the bone up to its stop, and left in place. All alignments are confirmed. The 6-mm drill is then drilled through the lower hole in the guide up to its collar (Fig. 4.23). Both drills and all instruments are removed. The intramedullary rod can be removed with the universal removal hook.

It is possible to use the extramedullary guide instead of the intramedullary rod. If this is done the patella must be retracted laterally so that it does not impinge on the drill guide.

Figure 4.23

Femoral saw cut

The femoral saw guide is inserted into the drilled holes and tapped home (Fig. 4.24)[2].

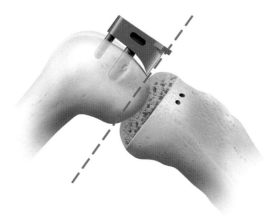

Figure 4.24

Using the 12-mm broad oscillating saw blade[1], the posterior facet of the femoral condyle is excised (Fig. 4.25). Care must be taken to avoid damage to the MCL and the ACL and to ensure that the cut is exactly in line with the guide.

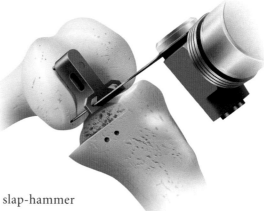

The saw guide is removed with the slap-hammer extractor taking care not to distort the drill holes.

There is now good access to the back of the joint and any remnants of the medial meniscus should be removed. We generally leave a small cuff of meniscus medially to protect the MCL from damage. We completely remove the posterior horn of the meniscus.

Figure 4.25

First milling of the condyle

Measurement with feeler gauges and spigots

The numbers marked on the feeler gauges and the meniscal bearings represent their least thickness in millimetres.

The scale of numbers of the spigots is in 1-mm steps, in inverse ratio to the thickness of their flanges.

The spigots are used as described below.

- First milling

  The 0 spigot is always used first. It is designed to remove sufficient bone to allow the femoral component to seat. It establishes a 'zero' from which succeeding measurements are made.

- Second milling

  The spigots (numbered 1–7) allow bone to be removed in measured quantities (in mm) from the level of the first mill cut. The number 3 spigot removes 3 mm, the number 4, 4 mm, etc.

- Subsequent milling

  If the last spigot used was a number 3, a number 4 spigot will remove a further 1 mm of bone (i.e. a total of 4 mm since the first milling). If the last spigot used was a number 4, a number 5 spigot is required to remove 1 mm of bone (i.e. a total thickness of 5 mm since the first milling).

Therefore the spigot number represents the total thickness of bone it removes from the level of the first (0) mill cut.

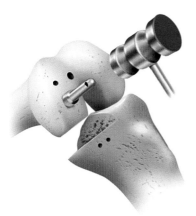

Insert the 0 spigot (the one with the thickest flange) into the large drill hole and tap it home until its flange abuts against the bone (Fig. 4.26).

Figure 4.26

By extending the knee to about 60° and retracting the soft tissues, the spherical mill can be manoeuvred onto the spigot (Fig. 4.27) and into the wound so that its teeth touch the bone (Fig. 4.28). To avoid trapping soft tissues, do not start the mill until it is touching bone.

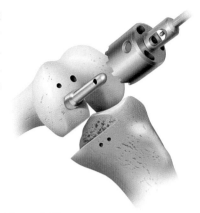

Figure 4.27

When milling, push firmly in the direction of the axis of the spigot, taking care not to tilt the tool. Mill until the cutter will not advance further. If in doubt continue to mill; there is no risk of over-milling.

Rarely, the defect on the femur is very deep and there may be a risk of removing too much bone at this first milling. Under these circumstances, milling should cease 2 mm before reaching the stop, as seen through the window in the mill.

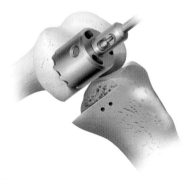

Figure 4.28

Remove the mill and the spigot and trim off the bone protruding from the posterior corners of the condyle which lie outside the periphery of the cutting teeth (Fig. 4.29). These corners of bone should be removed tangentially to the milled surface, and not parallel to the posterior surface. Also remove the small collar of bone that lay beneath the flange of the spigot and escaped milling.

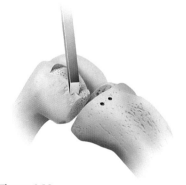

Figure 4.29

Equalizing the 90° and 20° flexion gaps

With the leg in 90° of flexion, insert the tibial template and apply the femoral trial component to the milled condyle, tapping it home with the femoral impactor angled 45° to the femoral axis.

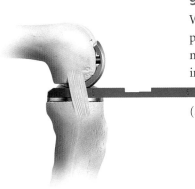

Figure 4.30

(a) The 90° flexion gap is now carefully measured with the feeler gauges (Fig. 4.30). (The tibial preparation has already ensured that the gap is wide enough to accept at least the 4-mm gauge.) The gauge thickness is correct when natural tension in the ligaments is achieved. Under these circumstances the feeler gauge will slide in and out easily but will not tilt.

(b) The gauge is removed. It is important to remove the feeler gauge before extending the knee because, at this stage, the extension gap is always narrower than the flexion gap. **If it is left in place, the gauge may stretch or avulse the ligaments as the knee extends.**

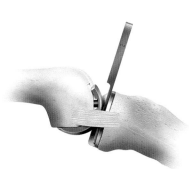

Figure 4.31

(c) The 20° flexion gap is measured next (Fig. 4.31) with the bone in 20° of flexion not full extension. (In full extension, the posterior capsule is tight and its influence gives a false undermeasurement.) The 20° flexion gap is almost always less than 4 mm, so either the thin plastic or metal feeler gauges are used to measure it. If the 1-mm gauge cannot be inserted, the gap is assumed to be 0 mm.

The formula for balancing the 90° and 20° flexion gaps is:

90° flexion gap (mm) − 20° flexion gap (mm) = thickness of bone to be milled from the femur (mm)
= spigot number to be used.

For instance, if the 90° flexion gap measures 5 mm and the 20° flexion gap 2 mm, then the amount of bone to be milled is 3 mm. To achieve this, insert a 3 spigot and mill until the cutter will advance no further

After each milling it is necessary to remove the bone left at the posterior corners of the condyle (see Fig. 4.29) and the collar of bone left under the flange of the spigot. The reference for the spigot will not be lost as its tip continues to reference off the bottom of the drill hole.

Confirming equality of the 90° and 20° flexion gaps

With the tibial template and the femoral trial component in place, re-measure the gaps. They will usually be found to be the same (Figs. 4.32 and 4.33).

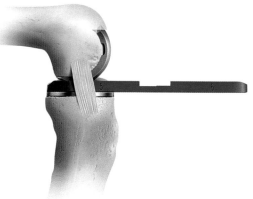

Figure 4.32

If the 20° flexion gap is still smaller than the 90° flexion gap, remove more bone with the mill. This can be done, 1 mm at a time, by using the sequence of spigots. (In the example above, a further 1 mm of bone could be removed by using a 4 spigot.) Do not hammer the spigot in if the collar of bone around the hole has been removed as this will destroy the reference at the bottom of the hole. The surgeon should look through the window in the mill to determine when milling is complete.

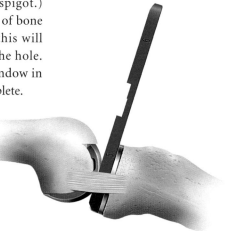

Usually the gaps are balanced with a 3 or 4 spigot.

Figure 4.33

Preventing impingement

Final preparation of the femur requires trimming of the femoral condyle anteriorly and posteriorly to avoid impingement of bone against the bearing in full extension and full flexion.

Anteriorly, a chisel is used to remove about 5 mm of bone to provide at least 3 mm clearance for the front of the bearing in full extension (Fig. 4.34).

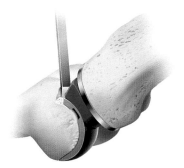

Figure 4.34

The femoral trimming guide is applied to direct the posterior osteophyte chisel (Fig. 4.35) so that it detaches all the osteophytes. The guide and osteophytes are removed, and a finger is inserted to confirm that the clearance is complete.

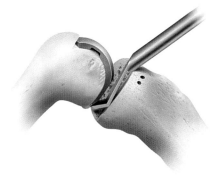

Figure 4.35

Final preparation of the tibial plateau

The tibial plateau is examined to ensure that there are no large marginal osteophytes medially. If there are, they should be removed, taking care not to damage the MCL.

The tibial template is inserted and located with its posterior margin flush with the posterior tibial cortex. The universal removal hook, passed over the posterior margin of the component and the tibia, facilitates this. The sizing of the tibial component is checked and altered if necessary. **Medially** and **posteriorly** the edge of the component should be aligned with the cortex or should overhang by up to 2 mm. If these two criteria are satisfied it does not matter if (as is usual) the front edge of the implant does not reach to the anterior cortex.

The template is fixed with the tibial template nail (Fig. 4.36). Cuts 1 cm deep are made with a reciprocating saw blade along both sides of the slot in the tibial template. A third oblique saw cut in the slot facilitates removal of eburnated bone. Take care that the cuts are no deeper than 1 cm.

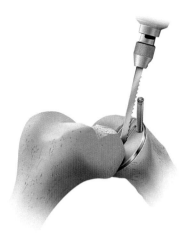

Figure 4.36

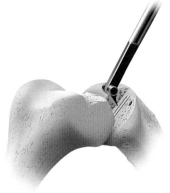

After removing the template, the groove is excavated to the correct depth by scooping out the bone with the blade of the tibial gouge, taking care not to damage the anterior and posterior cortices (Fig. 4.37). The safest way to prepare the back of the groove is to feel the posterior cortex with the pick and then move it forwards 5 mm before pushing it down into the bone and drawing it forward to empty the slot.

Figure 4.37

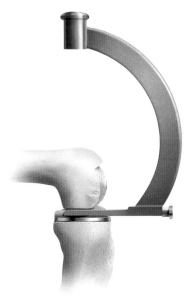

The tibial trial component is inserted and tapped home with the tibial impactor (Fig. 4.38).

Ensure that it is flush to the bone and that its posterior margin extends to the back of the tibia. Note where the anterior edge of the implant lies relative to the tibia so that the definitive component can be cemented in the same place.

During impaction of the tibial implant, the assistant should support the leg with a hand under the foot to avoid damage to the knee ligaments. Only a light hammer should be used, to avoid the risk of plateau fracture. If the component does not seat fully, it should be removed and the keel slot cleaned out again.

Figure 4.38

Trial reduction

Insert the tibial and femoral trial components, ensuring that they are fully seated by tapping them home with the appropriate impactors (Figs 4.39 and 4.40).

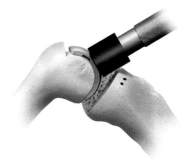

Figure 4.39

Insert a trial meniscal bearing of the chosen thickness (Fig. 4.41). (It is only at this stage that a trial bearing is used. Previously, feeler gauges have been used to measure the gaps because they do not stretch the ligaments. The meniscal bearings have a 3-mm high posterior lip which, after multiple insertions, may stretch the ligaments.)

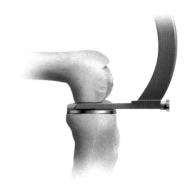

Figure 4.40

With the bearing in place, the knee is manipulated through a full range of movements to demonstrate stability of the joint, security of the bearing, and absence of impingement. The thickness of the bearing should be such as to restore the ligaments to their natural tension so that, when a valgus force is applied to the knee, the artificial joint surfaces distract a millimetre or two. This test should be done with the knee in 20° of flexion. In full extension the bearing will be firmly gripped because of the tight posterior capsule.

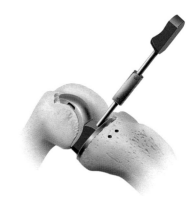

Figure 4.41

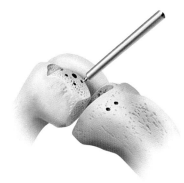

Figure 4.42

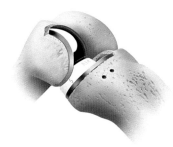

Figure 4.43

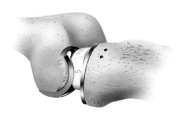

Figure 4.44

Cementing the components

The femoral and tibial surfaces are roughened by multiple small drill holes made with the cement key drill (Fig. 4.42). It is particularly important to make holes in areas of eburnated bone on the femur and tibia and in the posterior surface of the femur.

The components are fixed with two separate mixes of cement.

1. The tibial component A small amount of cement is placed on the tibial bone surface and flattened to produce a thin layer. The component is inserted and pressed down, first posteriorly and then anteriorly, so that excess cement is squeezed out at the front. The tibial impactor is used (with a small hammer) to complete the insertion. Excess cement is removed from the margins of the component using a small curette. A dissector is passed over the edge of the component to ensure that no soft tissue is under the component. If there is soft tissue it must be pulled out. The femoral trial component is then inserted and, with the knee flexed 45°, the appropriate feeler gauge is inserted to pressurize the cement. **During setting, the leg is held in 45° flexion and is compressed**. Do not fully extend the leg as pressure in this position may tilt the tibial component anteriorly. When the cement has set, remove the feeler gauge and the trial femoral component and look carefully for extruded cement. The flat plastic probe is made to slide along the tibial articular surface, feeling for cement at the edges, particularly posteriorly.

2. The femoral component From the second mix, a little cement is pushed into the large femoral drill hole and the concave surface of the femoral component is filled with cement. The loaded component is applied to the condyle and impacted with the punch held at 45° to the long axis of the femur. Excess cement is removed from the margins with a small curette and, with the knee flexed 45°, the appropriate feeler gauge is inserted to pressurize the cement. **During setting, the leg is compressed**

in 45° flexion as above. When the cement has set the feeler gauge is removed. The medial and lateral margins of the component are cleared of any extruded cement. The posterior margin of the implant cannot be seen, but it can be palpated with a curved dissector.

As the components may not have seated down fully the trial bearings are inserted again to select the ideal bearing thickness.

The reconstruction is completed by snapping the chosen bearing into place (Figs. 4.43 and 4.44).

Closure of the wound follows.

Notes

1. We strongly recommend the blade manufactured by Synvasive Technology Inc, Eldorado Hills, California, USA.

2. Most instrument sets provide a plane femoral saw guide, but slotted guides are available.

Instruments

1. Tibial saw guide assembly:
   (a) upper shaft, right
   (b) upper shaft, left
   (c) lower shaft
   (d) ankle yoke
   (e) ankle strap
2. MCL retractor
3. Headless nail
4. Headed nail
5. Nail puller
6. Intramedullary alignment rod (300 mm long)
7. Intramedullary alignment rod (200 mm long)
8. Rod pusher
9. Universal removal hook

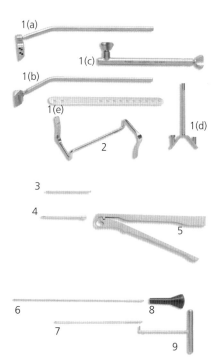

10. Femoral impactor
11. Drill (4 mm diameter)
12. Drill (6 mm diameter)
13. Slotted femoral saw guide
14. Plane femoral saw guide
15. Trial femoral component
16. Femoral drill guide
17. Metal feeler gauges (1, 2, and 3 mm thick)
18. Trial bearing (3 mm thick)
19. Trial bearings (4–9 mm thick)
20. Feeler gauges (3–9 mm thick)
21. Spherical mill
22. Spigots (0–7)

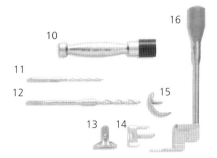
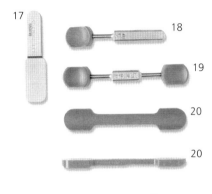
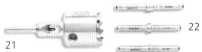
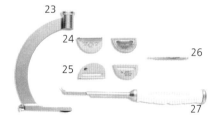
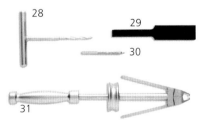

23. Tibial impactor
24. Trial tibial components
25. Tibial templates
26. Tibial template nail
27. Tibial groove gouge
28. Awl (5 mm diameter)
29. Plastic probe
30. Cement key drill
31. Slap-hammer extractor
32. Posterior osteophyte chisel
33. Femoral trimming guide

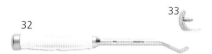

Postoperative management and radiography

Pain control

In the early postoperative period good pain control is essential. Regimes of pain management appropriate for total knee replacement may not be suited to the very rapid mobilization that is possible after UKA through a minimally invasive approach.

Intraoperative local anaesthesia

We have found that the most useful technique is a local anaesthetic block injected into the damaged tissues in the last stages of the operation. Our technique was developed from that of Kohan L and Kerr D (personal communication).

Ropivicane 300 mg, ketorolac 30 mg, and epinephrine 0.5 mg are made up to a total volume of 100 ml with normal saline and put in two 50-ml syringes. Before the components of the implant are cemented, the mixture is injected through a 19 gauge spinal needle into any tissue that was damaged during the operation. This is done methodically so that no area is missed, with particular attention being paid to the posterior capsule and the margins of the incision in the quadriceps muscle. The skin is infiltrated up to 3 cm from the margins of the wound and 10 ml is reserved until the end of the procedure to inject around the drain site.

This usually results in very little pain when the patient wakes from the anaesthetic, allowing immediate resumption of knee flexion and walking. Occasionally, however, the local anaesthetic is slow to work and patients awake with severe pain. Pain immediately after the operation can be more reliably avoided by regional nerve blocks given at the beginning of the procedure. They have the additional advantage of minimizing the dose of general anaesthetic required, which helps with more rapid recovery. However, femoral and sciatic nerve blocks with bupivicaine, and epidural anaesthesia, may have motor effects that delay mobilization. Therefore we now use prilocaine nerve blocks or a short-acting spinal anaesthetic. The effects of these have usually worn off 2–3 hours after the operation when the patients start to walk.

Severe pain may occur on the second day when all these drugs have ceased to act. This can be controlled by instilling local anaesthetic into the joint through a fine (epidural) catheter inserted into the knee before wound closure. The catheter should be fitted with a bacterial filter to minimize the risk of infection. The morning after surgery, 20 ml of 0.5 per cent bupivicaine is instilled into the joint. (If a suction drain was used it should be clamped.) The catheter (and drain) are then removed. This can provide good pain relief for a further 24 hours.

In addition to the local anaesthetic, we use high doses of enteral anti-inflammatory drugs with a gastroprotective agent such as ranitidine.

Blood loss

The amount of blood lost is insignificant and transfusion is not required. We routinely use a thigh tourniquet for the operation. Occasionally, in a patient with a compromised circulation, we have carried out the procedure without a tourniquet, but it is much more difficult.

We insert a vacuum drain into the joint at the end of the operation. It is placed in the lateral gutter of the knee so that it does not interfere with early knee flexion. Occasionally, if a drain is not used, there are acute haemarthroses in the postoperative period that delay rehabilitation.

The drain is removed the morning after surgery (or 4–5 hours postoperatively if the patient is to go home on the day of operation).

Rehabilitation

Range of motion

Patients recuperate from UKA more rapidly and more predictably than after TKA and do not require formal exercise regimes to recover knee movement. Vigorous exercises may even be counterproductive by making the knee more painful and swollen.

On the day of the operation, while the local anaesthetic block is providing good pain relief and the drain is in place, most patients can easily flex the knee to 90°. Thereafter, the joint tends to become more swollen, pain relief is less complete, and flexion is more difficult. Exercises to encourage flexion at this stage may make the knee worse, and patients should be allowed to limit knee movement within the range that is comfortable.

By the end of the first week, pain and swelling subside. Motion is gradually regained in succeeding weeks, usually recovering to what it was preoperatively after a month and often improving further thereafter.

Ambulation

Most patients start to walk about 2–3 hours after the operation. Early walking seems to improve the pain relief. If there is quadriceps weakness, splinting the knee may help.

Early discharge

Because they recover rapidly it is possible to discharge patients from hospital early. Repicci and Eberle [1] were able to treat 80 per cent of their patients with less than 24 hours in hospital.

We undertook a randomized study, within the setting of the UK National Health Service, to compare the effect of discharge on the day after operation with our routine practice (which is discharge on day 4 or 5) [2]. In appropriately selected patients, discharge on the day after operation did not prejudice the speed of recovery or increase the incidence of complications. However, it did result in a significant cost saving [3]. For patients to be discharged so early they must be relatively fit and live locally, and it is necessary to establish a support system so that patients can telephone if they have problems and be readmitted if necessary.

Duration of recovery

The early rapid recovery of function after UKA tends to slow down in later weeks. Often, at 6 weeks, patients are disappointed that they still have symptoms (although these are usually less severe than those experienced at the same stage after TKA). Therefore we warn patients before discharge that their rapid rate of recovery may not continue and that they may still have some pain medially (and some numbness laterally) at 2–3 months. Swelling of the knee is also likely to persist, with stiffness and restriction of extension and flexion for the next few months. These symptoms gradually improve over a period as long as a year.

Postoperative radiology

Good postoperative radiographs are necessary as a baseline for comparison with later films and to allow 'quality control' of the surgical technique.

For these purposes, the standard methods of aligning the X-ray beam are not sufficiently accurate, nor repeatable enough. To assess the positions of the two metal components, the X-ray beam must be centred on one component and aligned with it in two planes. The resulting projection of the other component can then be used to deduce their relative positions.

In the **anteroposterior projection**, the patient lies supine on the X-ray table and the leg and the X-ray beam are manipulated under fluoroscopic control until the tibial

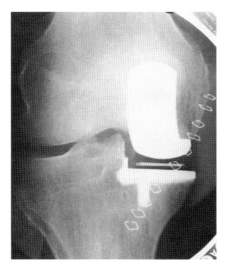

Figure 5.1 Fluoroscopically centred anteroposterior radiograph.

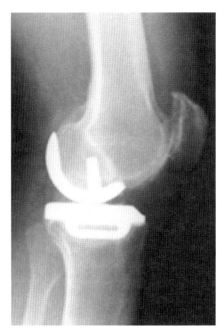

Figure 5.2 Fluoroscopically centred lateral radiograph.

component appears exactly end-on in silhouette, and the radiograph is then taken (Fig. 5.1). In this projection, the alignment of the beam with the flat orthogonal surfaces (horizontal tray and vertical lateral wall and keel) allows great accuracy and reproducibility.

In the **lateral projection**, the patient lies supine on the couch with the knee flexed 20°–30°. The fluoroscope is rotated through 90° so that the X-ray beam is parallel to the floor and centred on the femoral component (Fig. 5.2). (The tibial implant is not so useful in this projection as it offers no vertical surface and its horizontal surface is obscured by its lateral wall.) Therefore the lateral projection is not as precise or as reproducible as the anteroposterior projection.

Radiographs taken in this way can be repeated at any time interval in the knowledge that (at least in the anteroposterior films) the projections of the tibial component are always the same. Therefore small changes in the relationships of the components to one another and to the bones can be detected. Furthermore, because the X-ray beam is parallel to the tibial plateau, the state of its bone/implant interface is always reliably imaged. Without properly aligned postoperative films for comparison, later radiographs are difficult, or impossible, to interpret.

Quality control: component position and the interfaces

The postoperative radiographs can be used to measure the accuracy with which the prosthesis has been implanted.

Tibial component

On the anteroposterior projection, the component should appear at approximately 90° (±5°) to the tibial axis (Fig. 5.3). The medial margin should always reach to the medial tibial cortex and may overhang a little (no more than 2 mm in case it causes soft tissue irritation). The bone–implant interface should show a thin complete cement layer with a few millimetres penetration into the bone. (Cement penetration is deeper laterally and around the keel than medially, where the subchondral bone is less porous.) If the vertical

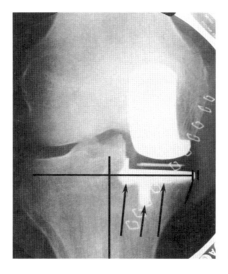

Figure 5.3 See text for details.

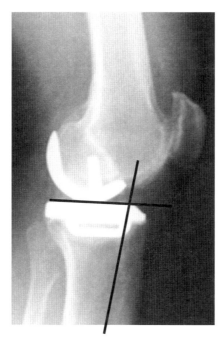

Figure 5.4 See text for details.

saw cuts have been made too deep (increasing the risk of fracture), they may be outlined by opaque cement or show up as vertical lucent lines. (The horizontal saw cut may have undermined the tibial eminence laterally, but this has no serious consequences.)

On the lateral projection, the component should slope downwards and backwards at about 7° to the tibial axis (Fig. 5.4). The posterior edge of the component should reach to the posterior cortex but should not overhang more than 1 mm. More overhang than this implies that the posterior cortex was damaged when the groove for the keel was excavated.

Femoral component

On the anteroposterior projection, the femoral component usually has the appearance of a 'bucket seat' (Fig. 5.5), with the component internally rotated about 15° relative to the tibia. To explain this, it must be remembered that when the component was implanted on the femur the knee was flexed to 90°. For the radiograph, the knee has been fully extended, a movement that is accompanied by obligatory internal rotation of the femur on the tibia (by about 15°).

On the lateral projection, the fixation peg should be parallel to the long axis of the femur (Fig. 5.6). A 'flexed' position of the peg implies diminished articular surface available in extension; an 'extended' position means there will be too little surface for full flexion.

The bone–implant interfaces of the femoral component are not as readily seen as those of the tibial implant. The inner surface of the inferior facet of the femoral component is concave, so that interface is hidden by the metal. The only interface that is readily imaged is at the flat posterior facet. If the radiographic technique has resulted in a true lateral silhouette, that interface is visible. It should present a thin parallel-sided layer of cement, with shallow penetration of the dense femoral bone. The central peg of the implant should appear solidly cemented in the drill hole.

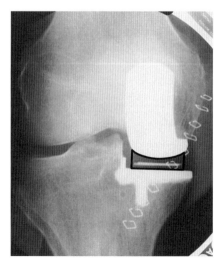

Figure 5.5 See text for details.

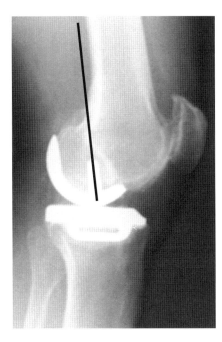

Figure 5.6 See text for details.

Meniscal bearing

On the anteroposterior projection, the mediolateral position of the bearing on the tibial plateau is deduced from the position of the femoral component (Fig. 5.5). The bearing should lie with its lateral edge 2–3 mm away from the wall of the tibial implant. Its position is explained by remembering that the bearing was positioned 1 mm from the wall with the knee flexed 90°. The radiograph is taken with the knee extended, and extension causes the bearing to glide not only forward on the plateau but also 1–2 mm medially, away from the wall (Chapter 3, Fig. 3.17). This medial displacement is probably associated with the obligatory internal rotation of the femur referred to above.

On the lateral projection, the anteroposterior position of the bearing on the tibial component is deduced from the radiological markers within it and from the position of the femoral component.

Impingement

The proper function of the OUKA depends upon the unimpeded freedom of the bearing to translate on the surfaces of the fixed components. The limits to its movement must be set by tension in the cruciate and collateral ligaments, not by impingement against retained osteophytes or fragments of cement.

The lateral projection may reveal retained posterior osteophytes on the femur or extruded cement at the back of the tibial component, either of which may impinge on the posterior edge of the bearing in flexion (Fig. 5.7).

Impingement anteriorly, due to inadequate removal of femoral bone from in front of the component, is the most frequent finding in retrieved bearings, but radiographs do not show this site well.

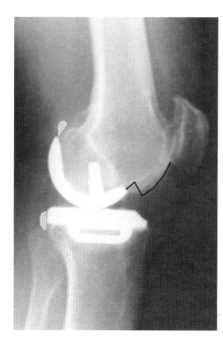

Figure 5.7 The sites of possible impingement of the bearing are indicated.

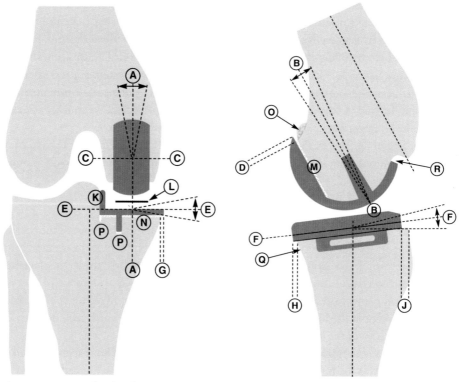

Figure 5.8 See text for details.

Scoring the postoperative radiographs

The diagrams in Figure 5.8 itemize the radiographic features described above. If the steps of the operation have been exactly followed, the postoperative appearances will be as shown in them.

Radiolucent lines

Radiolucent lines

The geometry of the tibial implant and the method of fluoroscopically controlled radiography that we have employed to image it have provided abundant evidence of the X-ray appearances of the bone/cement/implant interface under that component. The radiolucent "line" seen on a radiograph is the image of a thin layer of relatively lucent material that can only be seen if the X-ray beam is parallel to it. The degree of accuracy required cannot be regularly achieved without the use of screened alignment (Fig. 5.9).

The almost ubiquitous appearance of radiolucency beneath the tibial components of the Oxford Knee (Phase 1) when using the fluoroscopic technique was reported in 1984 [4]. A radiolucent line was observed under at least one of the tibial components in 77 of 80 knees (96 per cent) in which radiodense cement had been used. Most of the radiolucencies were incomplete. The most common site was medial to the keel in the medial implants and lateral to the keel in the lateral implants. Radiolucency was also common

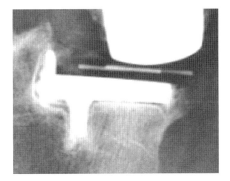

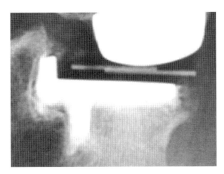

Figure 5.9 Two radiographs of the same knee taken on the same day. In the lower film the X-ray beam was tilted 2°, and the complete radiolucent line beneath the medial part of the plateau has disappeared.

around and under the keel. The radiolucent line was usually no more than 1 mm thick and none exceeded 3 mm.

The radiodense line

A striking feature of the radiographs was the presence of a thin radiodense line in the bone immediately adjacent to the radiolucences. It was present in all but three of the 77 knees with radiolucent lines. It was also present, and more readily seen, in all the 11 knees in which the components had been fixed with radiolucent cement (precluding the demonstration of the radiolucent line, the presence of which was inferred). In all these knees, a thin bone shell completely surrounded both tibial components, and the bone trabeculae could be seen inserting into it, as they do into the normal subchondral bone plate (Fig. 5.10).

Time of appearance

The radiolucent and the radiodense lines appeared at the same time, usually between 6 and 12 months after the arthroplasty. Once developed, they did not progress.

Natural history

Although the study referred to above was of bicompartmental Phase 1 Oxford prostheses (and some prototype implants), our subsequent experience has confirmed nearly all the conclusions drawn from it. The incidence in unicompartmental replacement with the Phase 2 and 3 implants is somewhat lower (75 per cent) than that mentioned above which referred to knees not compartments. No correlation has ever been found between clinical symptoms and the presence of radiolucency, and Röntgen stereometric analysis studies have shown no association with the rate of subsidence of the tibial component.

In a study of 26 knees examined radiographically 1 year and 10+ years after OUKA (Phases 1 and 2), 21 had partial or complete radiolucent lines around the tibial implant

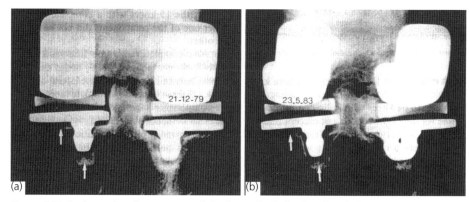

Figure 5.10 Radiographs of a prototype Oxford prosthesis fixed with radiolucent cement, taken (a) 1 year and (b) 5 years after implantation, showing the radiodense line surrounding both tibial components. (Reproduced with permission and copyright © of the British Editorial Society of Bone and Joint Surgery [Tibrewal SB, Grant KA, Goodfellow JW, The radiolucent line beneath the tibial components of the Oxford Meniscal Knee) *J Bone Joint Surg [Br]* 1984; **66-B**: 523–528].)

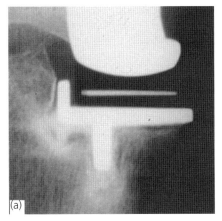

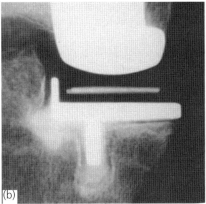

Figure 5.11 Physiological radiolucent and radiodense lines at (a) 1 year and (b) 10 years after implantation.

(Fig. 5.11) [5]. All but one were ≤1 mm thick. Only two had progressed between the early and late reviews, and only one of these was 2 mm thick.

Berger *et al.* [6] reported an incidence of 49 per cent partial or complete radiolucency around the tibial component of the Miller–Galante unicompartmental implant at 3–7 years review. None of them progressed after the third year and there was no instance of loosening of a component. The radiographs were not screened for alignment, which may explain the lower incidence.

Significance

We conclude that radiolucent lines around the tibial component of the OUKA are the rule not the exception, and that the radiographic technique mainly determines how frequently they are observed. They are probably as common around the femoral component, but are more difficult to demonstrate there. They do not appear to be the cause of symptoms nor evidence of loosening of the component. Therefore we refer to the radiographic appearances described above as 'physiological radiolucency'. They can usually be distinguished from the pathological lucency that surrounds an infected or a loose component by thickness and the presence of the radiodense line. The physiological lucent line is almost always <2 mm thick and defined by a thin radiodense bone plate; the pathological lesion is thicker, and the margins of the radiolucent zone are characteristically ill defined.

References

1. Repicci JA, Eberle RW. Minimally invasive technique for unicondylar knee arthroplasty. *J South Orthop Soc* 1999; **8**: 20–7.

2. Beard DJ, Murray DW, Rees JL, Price AJ, Dodd CA. Accelerated recovery for unicompartmental knee replacement: a feasibility study. *Knee* 2002; **9**: 221–4.

3. Shakespeare D, Jeffcote B. Unicondylar arthroplasty of the knee: cheap at half the price? *Knee* 2003; **10**: 357–61.

4. Tibrewal SB, Grant KA, Goodfellow JW. The radiolucent line beneath the tibial components of the Oxford meniscal knee. *J Bone Joint Surg [Br]* 1984; **66-B**: 523–8.

5. Weale AE, Murray DW, Crawford R, Psychoyios V, Bonomo A, Howell G, O'Connor J, Goodfellow JW. Does arthritis progress in the retained compartments after 'Oxford' medial unicompartmental arthroplasty? A clinical and radiological study with a minimum ten-year follow-up. *J Bone Joint Surg [Br]* 1999; **81-B**: 783–9.

6. Berger RA, Nedeff DD, Barden RM, Sheinkop MM, Jacobs JJ, Rosenberg AG, Galante JO. Unicompartmental knee arthroplasty. Clinical experience at 6- to 10- year follow up. *Clin Orthop* 1999; **367**: 50–60.

6

Results

The results of UKA can be gathered from three main sources: the reports of the National Registers, cohort studies, and prospective comparisons. In this chapter we attempt an overview of the results of UKA in general and OUKA in particular.

National registers

The Swedish Knee Arthroplasty Register (SKAR) was started in 1975, and several similar national registers have been set up more recently. Registers collect data at the time of primary surgery and when any revision operation is performed, ideally from all the surgeons in the country, so that cumulative revision rates (CRR) can be calculated. The large numbers provide narrow confidence limits, and subgroups large enough for statistical comparison. They are our best source of information on the epidemiology and demography of arthroplasty.

In SKAR, the CRR graphs are cut at 10 years (or earlier if the number at risk falls below 40). The results are updated annually and published on the Internet (http://www.ort.lu.se/knee/indexeng.html).

UKA versus TKA

Cumulative revision rate

The CRR for UKA in the decade 1993–2002 was about twice that for TKA for OA (Fig. 6.1). The graphs show that the patient's age at the time of surgery affected CRR similarly in both types of implant. The age profiles of the two were slightly different, with more of the UKA patients (30 per cent) under 65 years old.

Causes of failure

Figure 6.2 gives the percentage distribution of the indications for revision in UKA and TKA during the same period. In UKA, the three major causes of failure were loosening of a component, progression of arthritis to the retained compartments, and polyethylene wear.

The relatively low rate of infection in UKA means that, despite having a substantially higher CRR than TKA, '… the number of serious complications such as infection/arthrodesis/amputation is much less' [1].

Comparison of UKA models[1]

The registers are mainly consulted not for their demographic content but to compare the relative success of competing prostheses. Age, gender, and year of operation have been

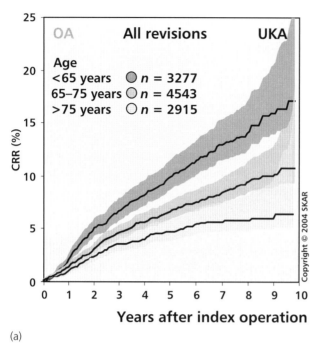

(a)

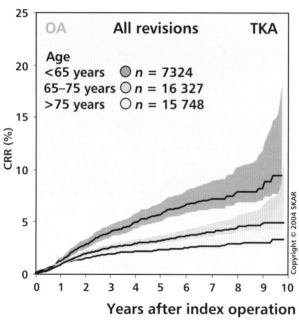

(b)

Figure 6.1 The differences in CRRs (1993–2002) in the age groups <65, 65–75, and >75 years for OA operated on with (a) UKA and (b) TKA. (Reproduced from the *Swedish Knee Arthroplasty Register Report 2004* with the permission of Dr O Robertsson.)

found to influence survival, and SKAR publishes Cox regression analyses for competing implants that take account of the effects of differences in their distribution. The results are then expressed as risk ratios. One implant is chosen as the index and is deemed to

Distribution of indications for revision (%) 1993–2002

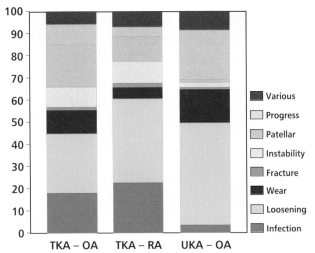

Figure 6.2 Distribution of indications for revision (per cent) for the period 1993–2002. (Reproduced from the *Swedish Knee Arthroplasty Register Report 2004* with the permission of Dr O Robertsson.)

have a risk ratio of 1.0. A Cox regression of, say, 1.2 implies a 20 per cent greater risk of revision.

Swedish Knee Arthroplasty Register 2004

Table 6.1 compares the UKA implants used in Sweden between 1993 and 2002. It shows their '95 per cent confidence intervals for the risk ratio with respect to revision'. The index implant was the Link Uni, the most widely used in Sweden. The implants shown in black type are those for which the risk of revision was not significantly different from that of the index model. Those shown in red type had a significantly greater risk of revision than the index.

Australian Orthopaedic Association Joint Replacement Registry (AJRR) 2004

The other register to have published a similar comparison, the Australian Orthopaedic Association Joint Replacement Registry (AJRR) [2], covers a much shorter period (September 1999–December 2004). Table 6.2 (taken from this report) gives the 95 per cent confidence intervals of 'revisions per 100 component years' for the models of UKA used in Australia. The authors stated that 'the Allegretto and Preservation have a significantly different performance from that of the index group, a cohort of the three knee implants with the lowest revision rates' (Miller-Galante, Repicci and Unix).

Cohort studies

The results of joint arthroplasty can also be evaluated from outcome studies of cohorts of patients, usually treated by one or a few surgeons. The predictive value of cumulative survival estimates based on cohort studies is diminished by incomplete follow-up and by too few subjects at risk in the later years [3,4]. Credibility is enhanced if other surgeons who employ the same selection criteria and have similar expertise in the use of the device report similar results.

Table 6.1 95% confidence intervals for the risk ratio with respect to revision (SKAR 2004)[1]

	OA/UKA	
	n	**95% CI**
Link Uni[a]	4356	Reference
Miller–Galante	1723	0.96–1.63
Marmor–Richards	1076	1.13–1.79
Brigham	687	0.89–1.60
Duracon	599	1.03–1.89
PFC	580	1.46–2.55
Oxford	572	0.90–1.80
Genesis	366	0.65–1.86
St Georg	290	0.46–1.24
Allegretto	255	0.85–2.05
Repicci	198	1.31–2.92
Other	31	
Gender (reference men)		0.89–1.21
Age (per year)		0.95–0.96
Year of operation (per year)		0.94–1.02

The Cox regression adjusts for difference in gender, age, and year of operation. Implants in red type had a significantly greater risk of revision than the index.

[a]Link Uni is the reference in UKA.

(Data reproduced from the *Swedish Knee Arthroplasty Register Report 2004* with the permission of Dr O Robertsson.)

Table 6.2 Unicompartmental primary knee procedures requiring revision (AJRR 2004)[1]

Unicompartmental	Number revised	Total number	Percentage revised	Observed 'component' years	Revisions per 100 observed 'component' years	Exact 95% CI
Allegretto Uni Knee	53	1051	5.0	1604	3.3	2.48–4.32
Genesis	11	478	2.3	497	2.2	1.10–3.96
Miller–Galante	23	965	2.4	1403	1.6	1.04–2.46
Oxford 3	155	4334	3.6	6553	2.4	2.01–2.77
PFC Sigma	9	137	6.6	348	2.6	1.18–4.91
Preservation	42	1028	4.1	1052	4.0	2.88–5.39
Repicci	23	1348	1.7	1888	1.2	0.77–1.83
Unix	14	708	2.0	1002	1.4	0.76–2.35
Others	19	778	2.4	601	3.2	1.90–4.94
Total	349	10 827	3.2	14 948	2.3	2.10–2.59

(Data reproduced with permission from the *Australian Orthopaedic Association National Joint Replacement Registry Annual Report 2004*.)

Table 6.3 Published cohorts of fixed bearing unicompartmental arthroplasties[1]

Year	Authors	Compartment	Prosthesis	Number	Survival rate (%) (95% CI)	
					10-year	**15-year**
1992	Capra and Fehring [32]	Medial/lateral	Marmor	52	94 (?)	–
1993	Heck et al.[33]	Medial/lateral	Marmor	294	91 (86–97)	–
1996	Cartier et al.[34]	Medial/lateral	Marmor	207	93 (81–100)	–
1998	Tabor and Tabor [35]	Medial/lateral	Marmor	67	84 (?)	79 (?)
1999	Squire et al. [36]	Medial/lateral	Marmor	140	89 (84–95)	87 (78–95)
1991	Neider [37]	Medial	St Georg	548	80 (?)	
1994	Weale and Newman [38]	Medial	St Georg	42	90 (?)	88 (?)
1997	Ansari et al. [39]	Medial	St Georg	461	87 (81–93)	
1991	Scott et al. [40]	Medial/lateral	Brigham	100	85 (67–99)	–
1998	Hasegawa et al. [41]	Medial	PCA	77	88 (?)	–
1998	Bert [42]	Medial	MBUKA	100	87 (?)	–
1999	Berger et al. [43]	Medial/lateral	Miller–Galante	62	98 (96–100)	–
2002	Argenson et al. [44]	Medial	Miller–Galante	160	94 (91–97)	–

? Confidence intervals not published.

(Data adapted from and reproduced with permission from Lippincott Williams & Wilkins from Price AJ, Svard U. Long-term Clinical Results of the Medial Oxford Unicompartmental Knee Arthroplasty. *Clin Orthop* 2005; **435**: 171–180.)

UKA versus TKA

Table 6.3 shows survival data from cohort studies of several models of UKA (all with fixed bearings) using revision for any cause as the endpoint [5]. Since there are few published survival tables, some of the numbers were deduced from survival curves and therefore are approximate.

When compared with TKA (Table 6.4), UKA generally has 6–7 per cent worse survival at 10 years, a difference similar to that reported by SKAR.

Comparison of UKA models

The Marmor, St Georg, and Miller–Galante UKAs achieved 90 per cent survival or better at 10 years in at least one cohort. Neither of the fixed-bearing UKAs with survival data up to 15 years (Marmor and St Georg) maintained their 90 per cent survival at that interval (Table 6.3).

Table 6.5 shows the results of the seven published cohorts of OUKA with 10-year survival rates. The combined data are from 1040 OUKAs performed by 11 surgeons. Of these, > 282 were at risk at 10 years and 26 at 15 years.

Prospective comparisons

Randomized controlled trials (RCTs), which are the established method of comparison in clinical medicine, are more difficult to organize in surgery, and many fewer surgical than medical treatments are based on such sound evidence. There is no published RCT with 10-year CRR for comparison of survival of UKA models.

Table 6.4 Published cohorts of total knee arthroplasties (endpoint is all-cause revision unless otherwise stated)

Year	Authors	Prosthesis	Number	Survival rate (%) (95% CI)	
				10-year	**15-year**
2001	Ritter *et al.* [45]	AGC	4583	99	99 (94–100)*
2000	Robertsson *et al.* [46]	Freeman–Samuelson	190	96 (90–100)	–
2001	Laskin [47]	Genesis (PCL retaining)	56	96 (?)	–
2001	Laskin [47]	Genesis (PCL sacrificing)	44	97 (?)	–
2001	Brassard *et al.* [48]	IB I	165	96 (92–100)b	–
2001	Brassard *et al.* [48]	IB II	160	98 (?)b	–
1995	Malkani *et al.* [49]	Kinematic	168	96 (93–99)	–
1996	Weir *et al.* [50]	Kinematic	208	92 (87–95)	–
2000	Berger *et al.* [51]	Miller–Galante I	172	84 (80–88)	–
2001	Berger *et al.* [52]	Miller–Galante II	109	100 (100–100)	–
1995	Colizza *et al.* [53]	Total condylar PS	165	98 (95–100)	–
1993	Ranawat *et al.* [54]	Total condylar	112	99 (?)	94 (?)
2001	Pavone *et al.* [55]	Total condylar	120	–	91 (?)
1999	Gill *et al.* [56]	Total condylar	72	99 (91–100)	99 (91–100)
2001	Rodriguez *et al.* [57]	Total condylar	220	100 (99–100)	95 (95–99)

? Confidence intervals not published.

*Revision of patella not counted as failure.

(Adapted and reproduced, with permission, from the DPhil thesis of AJ Price [23])

Emerson *et al.* [6] compared two cohorts of patients, all treated between 1986 and 1994, with either a fixed-bearing UKA (Brigham, 51 knees) or an OUKA Phase 2 (50 knees). The method of treatment was not randomized, but the preoperative profiles were similar in the two cohorts. The mean follow-up times were 6.1 (0.5–13.2) years and 6.8 (2–10.9) years, respectively. The mean postoperative Knee Society scores at review were 89.0 and 92.0, respectively, and the mean pain scores were 43.1 and 45.2, respectively. The cumulative survival at 11 years was 92 per cent for both implants.

Although these measurements showed no difference between the two models, there was a difference in the ways in which each failed. Of the eight fixed-bearing implants that were revised, four were for polyethylene wear and two for loosening of the tibial component. Of the seven OUKAs that were revised, none was for wear or tibial loosening, and four were for progression of arthritis in the lateral compartment. The authors also noted that the varus deformity was corrected to more nearly normal alignment by the OUKA and suggested that this placed increased stress on the lateral compartment.

Table 6.5 Published cohorts of Oxford unicompartmental arthroplasties

Year	Authors	Phase	Number	Mean follow-up (range) (years)	10-year survival (%)	95% CI	No. at risk	15-year survival (%)	95% CI	No. at risk
1998	Kumar and Fiddian [58]	2	83	5.6 (1–11)	85	78–92	?			
1998	Murray et al. [59]	1, 2	144	7.6 (6–14)	98	93–100	33			
2002	Emerson et al. [6]	2	50	6.8 (2–13)	92	–				
2004	Rajasekhar et al. [60]	2	135	5.8 (2–12)	94	84–97	22			
2005	Keys et al. [20]	2	40	7.5 (6–10)	100	–	6			
2005	Vorlat et al. [61]	2	149	5.5 (1–10)	84	(SE 6.9)	82			
2005	Price et al. [5]	1, 2, 3	439	(1–15)	93	89–99	139	93	84–100	26

Gleeson *et al.* [7] compared two cohorts of 47 OUKAs (Phase 3) and 57 St Georg Sled UKAs. The intention was to allot the patients randomly, but the protocol was not followed in 33 cases. Most of the operations were performed through a 'reduced incision', but this was difficult for the St Georg because of lack of appropriate instrumentation.

Clinical measurements were made at 2 years, although the mean follow-up time was 4 years (2.7–5.3). No survival statistics are given. Four OUKAs had been revised to TKAs, two for persistent pain, one for tibial subsidence, and one for tibial condyle fracture. Three St Georg Sleds were revised to TKAs, all for tibial loosening. Three OUKA bearings dislocated, all within 3 months of operation, and required surgical replacement but with a satisfactory outcome. The Bristol Knee score (BKS) and the Oxford Knee score were recorded at 2 years. The BKS pain score was significantly better for the St Georg (34.9 versus 30.7, $P = 0.013$).

The authors remarked that the complication rates were high in both cohorts. They attributed this to the technically demanding design of the OUKA, and to the 'basic' nature of the instrumentation of the St Georg which was inadequate to implant it through a small incision. The number of surgeons (and surgical trainees) who performed the operations was not reported.

Confalonieri *et al.* [8] described a cohort of 40 consecutive unicompartmental arthroplasties in which patients were randomly allotted either a fixed bearing UKA (Allegretto) or a mobile-bearing implant (AMC[1]). No statistically significant difference in any outcome measure was observed between the two implants. At an average follow-up of 5.7 years, one knee in the fixed-bearing group had been revised for unexplained persistent pain. None of the AMC implants had been revised and there had been no bearing dislocations. The authors claim this to be the only RCT to compare UKA designs.

Current practice: minimally invasive surgery with the OUKA

The foregoing results, in both the national registers and the cohort studies, were for operations which were almost all performed through an exposure like that used for TKA. Following the initiative of Repicci and Eberle [9], the number of UKAs performed through a small anterior arthrotomy, without dislocation of the patella, rapidly increased. By 2003, the proportion reported to SKAR had risen from 15 per cent in 1999 to 58 per cent. Some designs have been implanted more often by the minimally invasive method than others. For instance, by 2003, the great majority of the Miller–Galante UKAs and the OUKAs performed in Sweden were through a small incision but only about one-third of the St Georg/Link design were performed in this way [1].

Repicci and Eberle [9] compared the outcome of two sequential groups of 50 UKAs performed in 1992 and 1993: (1) by the open surgical approach, with dislocation of the patella; (2) through a small (8-cm) arthrotomy. In group 2 there was diminished blood loss intraoperatively and much quicker postoperative recovery. Their practice changed so that, subsequently, 80 per cent of UKA operations were performed as outpatient procedures.

Keys [10] reported the results of 10 OUKAs implanted through a small parapatellar incision using standard Phase 2 components and instrumentation. His patients recovered more rapidly than when the open approach was used, and with no loss of precision of implantation.

OUKA Phase 3

In 1998, to facilitate its use through a small incision, the OUKA instruments were slightly modified and a wider range of implant sizes was made available. The aim was to maximize the short-term benefits of reduced tissue damage while preserving the core aspects of the design.

Price *et al.* [11] reported on the first 40 OUKAs (10 Phase 2 and 30 Phase 3) implanted in Oxford by a single surgeon (DM) through a small incision and compared them with the last 20 Phase 2 prostheses implanted by the same surgeon using the open approach. The two cohorts followed one another with no break in sampling. Both cohorts were also compared with a group of 40 TKAs randomly chosen from operations performed under the care of the same surgeon during the same time period.

Speed of recovery

The 'time to recovery' was measured as the interval from operation to the achievement of the markers described by Keys [10]:

(1) straight-leg raising without quadriceps lag;

(2) knee flexion to 70°;

(3) walking, climbing, and descending stairs unaided.

Table 6.6 Criteria for accurate placement on postoperative radiographs

Femoral component

1. Parallelism between the posterior condylar bone cut and the flat non-articular surface of the femoral component
2. Flexion–extension alignment of the femoral component peg with the long axis of the femur
3. Position of the femoral component along the mediolateral axis of the knee
4. Defects in the femoral cement mantle

Tibial component

5. Relationship of the posterior margin of the tibial implant to the posterior margin of the tibial plateau
6. Variations from the ideal 7° posterior tilt in the lateral plane
7. Variations from the ideal horizontal alignment in the frontal plane
8. Defects in the cement mantle

Other

9. Retained osteophytes that could impinge on the bearing
10. Cement lying outside the interfaces

(Reprinted from *J Arthroplasty*, **Vol. 16**, Price AJ *et al.*, Rapid recovery after Oxford unicompartmental arthroplasty through a short incision, 970–6, copyright (2001), with permission from Elsevier.)

(These were the requirements for discharge applied by the physiotherapy department at the hospital.)

The time to recovery was shorter for OUKA than for TKA, and the use of a small incision instead of an open approach further reduced it to about 40 per cent of that for TKA.

Accuracy of placement

All the OUKAs in the study had postoperative radiographs aligned under fluoroscopic control. These were reviewed by two observers, on two occasions, who estimated the accuracy of surgical implantation by scoring 10 radiographic features (Table 6.6). (These observations could not be strictly blinded as the skin clips were visible on the radiograph and revealed the length of the incision.) There was no significant difference between the scores of the OUKAs implanted using the two different approaches.

Clinical outcome study of current practice with the OUKA

Pandit et al. [12] described the results of 688 OUKAs (Phase 3), all implanted by the minimally invasive approach by two surgeons (DM and CD) between 1998 and 2005. The indication for surgery was anteromedial OA in 667 and focal osteonecrosis in 21. Of these, 132 had been implanted for at least 5 years. The mean age of the patients at the time of surgery was 66.4 (33–88) years; 308 were men and 287 women. There were 93 bilateral procedures, 11 performed under one anaesthetic and the rest staged.

Cumulative survival rate

No patient was lost to follow-up. Nine knees had been revised. The reasons for revision were infection (four), unexplained persistent pain (two), and dislocation of the bearing (three). The cumulative survival at 7 years, when there were 34 knees at risk, was 97.3 per cent (95 per cent CI, 5.3).

Clinical measurements

Of the 132 knees that had been implanted for 5 years or more, 101 were examined at the 5-year follow-up clinic and had full clinical and radiological assessments and 25 were interviewed by telephone.

At five years, the mean AKSS (objective) was 91.2 (preoperative: 35.3) and the mean AKSS (functional) was 78.6 (preoperative: 49.6). Of the 101 knees reviewed clinically, 87 had an excellent AKSS, ten were good, two fair, and two poor. The mean OKS was 39.2 (preoperative: 18). The mean Tegner score was 2.6 (preoperative: 1.9). The mean preoperative flexion range of 115° improved to a mean 133° at five years.

Radiological measurements

The method described by Weale et al. [13] was used to assess progression of arthritis in the retained compartments. Fluoroscopically aligned anteroposterior and lateral radiographs taken 1 year after surgery were compared, in a blinded manner, with similar films taken at 5 years. The results are shown in Table 6.7.

Table 6.7 Radiological assessment of progression of arthritis in the retained compartments

Condition	Patellofemoral joint		Lateral compartment	
	Ahlback	Altman	Ahlback	Altman
Definitely worse	0	1	2	3
Possibly worse	3	2	3	2
Same	98	97	96	96
Possibly better	0	1	0	0
Definitely better	0	0	0	0

(Reproduced with permission and copyright © of the British Editorial Society of Bone and Joint Surgery [Pandit H, Jenkins C, Barker K, Dodd CAF, Murray DW. The Oxford medial unicompartmental knee replacement using a minimally-invasive approach. *J Bone Joint Surg* [Br] 2006; **88-B**; 54–60].)

'Surgical routine' and the learning curve

The term 'surgical routine', to include the expertise of the surgeon and the quality of perioperative management, was coined by Robertsson *et al.* [14] to explain the findings of a study of how the number of operations performed in an orthopaedic unit affected CRR. Data from SKAR (1986–1995) for three unicompartmental implants were used (Fig 6.3). The results from surgical units in which fewer than 23 UKA of all kinds were performed annually (group A) were compared with the results from the rest (group B). (The number 23 appears to be arbitrary.) The risk of revision in group A was 1.63 times (95 per cent CI, 1.41–1.89) that in group B. Comparison of these figures with the risk ratios for competing models (Table 6.1) suggests that the influence of the surgical routine on outcome is of the same order as choice of implant.

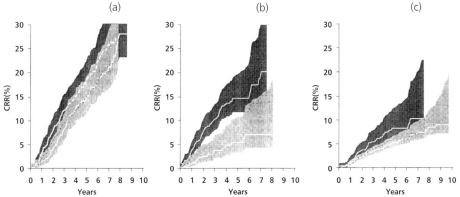

Figure 6.3 Graphs showing CRR for (a) 874 knees operated on using an implant with known mechanical and design problems (PCA), (b) 905 knees operated on using a technically demanding implant (OUKA) and (c) 4307 knees operated on using a commonly used implant (St Georg/Link). Lines represent the CRR and shaded areas the 95% confidence interval. The dark areas are surgical units performing a mean of less than 23 operations per annum; the light areas units doing more than 23 per annum. (Reproduced with permission and copyright © of the British Editorial Society of Bone and Joint Surgery [Robertsson O, Knutson K, Lewold S, Lidgren L. The routine of surgical management reduced failure after unicompartmental knee arthroplasty. *J Bone Joint Surg [Br]* 2001; **83-B**: 45–9]).

The PCA (Fig. 6.3(a)) had the worst survival in both groups. Its results were not significantly different between the groups and its poor performance was attributed to its '... inferior mechanical and design properties'.

The OUKA (Fig. 6.3(b)) had the best survival in group B but the risk of revision in group A was 3.07 times greater (95 per cent CI, 1.78–5.29). This dependence on who did the operation was attributed to its being a 'technically demanding' procedure. Whatever the explanation, the magnitude of the effect leaves no doubt about the importance of 'surgical routine'. The difference between the survival rate of the same implant in different hands (OUKA in groups A and B) was greater than the difference between the 'worst' and the 'best' of the 11 implants for which survival curves were published in SKAR 2004 (Table 6.1) [1].

The St Georg/Link Uni (Fig. 6.3(c)) had a survival similar to the OUKA in group B but its risk of revision was only 1.53 times (95 per cent CI, 1.10–2.12) greater in group A. This lesser dependence on surgical routine was attributed to its being more widely used and, by implication, less technically demanding.

The opinion has often been expressed that UKA is more demanding than TKA, with a smaller margin for error [15,16], and several authors have documented the phenomenon of the learning curve from their own experience.

Lindstrand et al. [17] reported the early results for a fixed-bearing UKA (Duracon) after it was first introduced into one centre specializing in arthroplasty and into four smaller centres with less previous experience of UKA. There was evidence of a learning curve in all the hospitals, but the combined results of the four smaller hospitals were not as good as those of the specialist centre. Seven of the total of eight revisions occurred among the first 10 operations performed in each hospital.

Jeer et al. [18] had a high early failure rate after introducing the LCS (mobile-bearing) UKA into their practice to replace the fixed-bearing device with which they had a long previous experience. They concluded that 'The introduction of a new system of UKA includes the risk of early failures due to surgeon error, even when a surgeon is competent in UKA ...' The errors referred to were not repeated in subsequent cases.

Rees et al. [19] reported the 1-year clinical outcome (American Knee Society score and Oxford Knee score) of the first 104 OUKAs (Phase 3) implanted through a small incision in Oxford. They showed that if the operating surgeon had done fewer than 10 such procedures, the results were significantly worse than if he or she had done more (mean AKSS 88 points and 95 points, respectively; $P < 0.03$) even though the beginners always operated under the direct supervision of an experienced surgeon.

However, Keys et al. [20] reviewed the first 40 consecutive OUKAs (Phase 2) performed by one surgeon at a district hospital where an average of eight were performed each year. The average follow-up was 7.5 (6–10) years, and no revision operations had been undertaken (10-year cumulative survival rate, 100 per cent). The authors claimed that their study did '... not support the observation that less number of these procedures performed each year correlate with a poorer outcome'. However, the surgeon had had previous experience of the operation elsewhere before he started his series at the small centre.

Life history of the OUKA

Since the introduction of the St Georg and Marmor prostheses there have been few innovations in UKA implant design. In 1982, the OUKA was a novelty, and it is still the only UKA to have a congruous mobile bearing. In 1987, its instrumentation also contrasted with the simple methodology then in use for UKA. It has now featured in SKAR reports and cohort studies for more than 20 years.

Swedish Knee Arthroplasty Register data

Lewold *et al.* [21] used SKAR data to compare the CRRs of 2365 Marmor UKAs and 699 OUKAs (Phase 1 and 2) in the period from 1983 (when the OUKA was introduced into Sweden) to 1992. During those 9 years, the OUKA was adopted by surgeons (we do not know how many) in 19 Swedish centres. Many early failures occurred, and at 2 years the failure rate was nearly five times that of the Marmor. At 7 years, the CRR for the OUKA (12.69 per cent) was twice that of the Marmor (6.33 per cent). At the two centres at which more than 100 procedures were performed, the results were said to be no better than the rest, and so the high failure rate was attributed to the design of the implant and not to surgical inexperience.

By 2000, however, the survival curves of the two designs had crossed and in 2003 (and 2004) the confidence intervals for the risk ratio for revision after OUKA were better than for the Marmor UKA and not significantly different from that of the index implant (see Table 6.1).

Cohort data

During almost the same time period (1983–2000), a prospective cohort study of OUKA implanted by three surgeons at one centre was also in progress in Sweden [22]. When its results were analysed by Price [23], the 10-year cumulative survival rate was 94 per cent and there was no significant difference between the 10-year survival rate for the Phase 1 design used until 1987 (96 per cent; CI, 4.1) and the Phase 2 design which was implanted thereafter (93 per cent; CI, 7.5).

Discussion

UKA versus TKA

The statistician needs a firm endpoint to construct survival tables, and 'revision' seems the best available. However, in comparing the two classes of implant it may introduce bias because the threshold for converting a UKA to a TKA is likely to be lower than for removing an unsatisfactory TKA and implanting another. Even if the number of unsatisfied patients was the same after both primary procedures, more UKAs might still be revised, first, because a TKA may seem, to the patient and the surgeon, the next rational therapeutic step and, second, because it is technically easier to do. The 2003 clinical survey of 35 000 patients in SKAR showed that about 6 per cent were 'unsatisfied' with the result of their knee replacement, and therefore were potential candidates for revision and susceptible to this bias. It is not possible to say how much of the observed

(6–7 per cent) difference in prosthetic survival between the two types of implant is due to the choice of revision as the endpoint, but its use makes it unlikely that UKA will ever rival TKA as measured by CRR.

Causes of revision

Polyethylene wear was the reported cause of about 15 per cent of UKA failures, but that may be an underestimate of its importance. The data presented by SKAR do not extend beyond 10 years, and polyethylene wear has most often been reported as a cause for revision in the second decade after implantation. It has not been reported as a cause of failure in OUKA (but see the section on bearing fractures in Chapter 7).

Wear may be under-reported as a cause of failure of fixed-bearing implants, because it can be the cause of loosening of a component. Marmor [24] reported that loosening was the eventual mode of failure of most of the thin (<7 mm) polyethylene components distorted by wear, and Christensen [15] observed, at revision operations, that '… whenever the components were firmly fixed, there was no wear of the tibial components while in the case of even slight looseness there was a considerable amount of wear'. Witvoet *et al.* [25] thought that polyethylene wear was the probable cause of loosening of the tibial component in 11 of 16 failed UKAs that they examined. The poor survival figures for fixed-bearing UKAs at 15 years suggests that they are not designed to last.

National registers versus cohort studies

> 'The model is the factor that generates the most interest and most often is related to the result after knee arthroplasty'. (SKAR 2004)

> 'The main purpose of the register is to function as a surveillance tool to identify inferior implants as early as possible'. (Norwegian Arthroplasty Register 2002)

National Registers have provided sound demographic information on the practice of arthroplasty, and a useful measure of the average (and regional) achievements of the participating surgeons. However, whether they are a good resource for the comparison of implants is more doubtful.

The outcome of UKA depends on patient selection and surgical expertise at least as much as on the design of the implant used. The registers collect little data on (and exert no control over) these two variables. Ironically, it seems that their predictive power may be least when it would prove most useful, i.e. during the period when an innovation is introduced into practice.

Patient selection

About 95 per cent of UKAs are done for 'osteoarthritis' of the knee [1], but within that broad category the registers collect no information on the precise pathology, such as the state of the ACL or the MCL, the extent of the cartilage erosions, or the degree of fixed deformity, on which outcome may mainly depend. Unlike TKA, UKA is appropriate in a minority of osteoarthritic knees, and its success depends upon its being implanted into the right minority.

Surgeon selection

Important as is patient selection, "surgeon selection" seems to have an even greater effect on the outcome of UKA. In using data from national registers to compare implants, the assumption is made that the results are achieved by the 'average' surgeon. If an implant, and the method of its insertion, have been standardized in a surgical community for many years, this may be a fair assumption, but it is not likely to be true of an innovation. The probable explanation for the gradual improvement in the SKAR results for OUKA compared with the Marmor UKA in Sweden over the period from 1983 to 2000 is the gradual diminution of the effects of the surgeons' learning curves. The results of the same implant, in the same country, in the hands of an expert were as good at the beginning of that period as at the end [23].

The study by Robertsson et al. [14] suggests that the overall statistical success of a given model depends upon the 'mix' of surgeons who performed it. A novel procedure may recruit learner surgeons to its use over many years, and it is the net expertise of all those employing it that determines its outcome in a national register. The study does not necessarily imply that continuous experience (i.e. >23 cases per annum) is necessary. With a small throughput, the learning curve may last longer, but once the expertise has been gained it may not require a large throughput to maintain it. Keys [10] achieved 100 per cent cumulative survival at 10 years performing an average of eight OUKAs per annum.

Some other observations support the suspicion that what the registers mainly measure is surgical expertise. Recently introduced UKA implants have generally had worse survival rates than established models. The fact that the SKAR has recorded no improvement, over the years, in the overall results of UKA was attributed in the 2004 report [1] to the effect of '... some newer models that have shown inferior results'. A similar statement was made 10 years earlier [26], but the procedures criticized then included the OUKA. This implant has since joined the establishment, but, in 2004, several of the implants with significantly high risk ratios for revision were 'newer models' (see Table 6.1).

There are other reasons to be cautious about the predictive power of the registers. The status of competing implants has often changed even in the short term. Of nine implants included in all three of the SKAR reports (in 2002, 2003, and 2004), five maintained the same status (relative to the index implant) throughout that period but the other four have been deemed, in at least one report, to be 'significantly' more (or less) likely to require revision than was reported in 2004 (Table 6.8).

Nor do the registers, so far, support one another. Comparison of the revision rates of the implants reported in both the Swedish and the Australian registers in 2004 (Tables 6.1 and 6.2) reveals no consensus, and suggests that something different from the effects of their design has been measured on one (or both) sides of the world.

Cohort studies

If the main problem with the national registers is their lack of control over surgical expertise, the problems with cohort studies are their relatively small patient numbers and the potential bias of their authors. These often are (or include) the inventor(s) of the

Table 6.8 Variations of risk of revision of competing implants in SKAR Reports 2002, 2003, and 2004

Implant	Year of SKAR report		
	2002	2003	2004
Marmor–Richards	↓	↓	↓
Miller–Galante	↓	↓	=
Oxford	↓	=	=
PFC	↓	↓	↓
Allegretto	↓	↓	=
Repicci	↓	↓	↓
Duracon	=	=	↓
Brigham	=	=	=
Genesis	=	=	=

The risk of revision of each implant is recorded as not significantly different from (=), or significantly worse than (↓) that of the index implant (Link Uni).

implant, or its enthusiastic champions, and even when there are no competing financial or professional interests, there may still be bias if the measurement of outcome is in the same hands that performed the operation.

However, surgical expertise and patient selection, the two variables that most confound the conclusions of the registers, can be better controlled. It can be assumed, for instance, that inventor surgeons will apply their own selection criteria and implant their own designs as well as possible, and thus that their results will represent the best that can be expected of the implant. Therefore comparison of outcome between such series should reflect the qualities of the implants. It also follows that if the results under these ideal circumstances are poor, the cause must lie with the implant. The mechanical deficiencies of the PCA prosthesis were first demonstrated not by the poor results achieved by the 'average surgeon', which could have had several explanations, but because not even its inventors reported good results.

The inadequacies of the national registers and the potential bias of the cohort studies point to the need for prospective comparisons of implant models before they reach the market, employing randomization of patients and blinded methods of measurement of outcome. However, most surgeons practice only one of several possible methods of treatment for a given clinical problem and cannot, without adverse bias, readily adopt an alternative method. A long learning period is often required to achieve a new expertise. The solution may lie in the organization of multi-centre, expertise-based RCTs as proposed by Deveraux et al. [27]. In such a trial, patients would be randomly allotted to different surgeons each with expertise in one of the competing implants. We know of no such comparison of unicompartmental replacements.

Comparison of fixed-bearing UKAs and OUKAs

Ten-year survival studies

The 2004 reports of SKAR and the AJRR reveal no significant differences between fixed-bearing UKAs and mobile-bearing OUKAs.

In the cohort studies, several fixed-bearing devices have achieved 10-year survival of 90 per cent or better in at least one study. The OUKA has achieved this in five of the seven published studies but with a wide range of results (84–100 per cent).

However, it is probable that the indications for surgery with the OUKA were different from those of the rest. Several fixed-bearing UKAs are recommended for use employing the widely accepted indications of Kozinn and Scott [28]. If strictly applied, these criteria have been found to identify 6 per cent [29] or 2 per cent [30] of osteoarthritic knees requiring surgery as suitable for UKA. As detailed in Chapter 2, we recommend many fewer limitations and have found our criteria to include about 30 per cent of osteoarthritic knees requiring surgery.

Fifteen-year survival studies

Neither of the fixed-bearing implants with longer term data (Marmor and St Georg) maintained their 90+ per cent survival to 15 years. The cohort of OUKA [5] with a 15-year survival of 93 per cent had 139 knees at risk at 10 years, none of which had failed in the succeeding 7 years. These figures are important because most patients live for longer than 10 years after their UKA. In two publications, in which the average age of the patients at surgery was 70 years, 66 per cent and 70 per cent, respectively, were still alive at the 10-year review [22,31]. The present trend is to use UKA in younger patients (see below), and so the 10-year results must be regarded as no more than mid-term. Failures in the second decade after surgery have very often been attributed to the direct or indirect effects of polyethylene wear, a mode of failure that occurs in the tibial components of all designs of fixed-bearing UKA but only rarely in congruous mobile bearings.

Current practice: minimally invasive surgery

In the hands of two experienced surgeons, each performing the operation about once a week, the 7-year cumulative survival of 688 OUKAs (Phase 3), all done through a minimally invasive incision, was not significantly different from that of Phase 1 and 2 procedures at the same interval [12]. Postoperative recovery was considerably quicker with the changed approach, and the accuracy of implantation, as measured on postoperative radiographs, was not prejudiced. The average range of postoperative movement was substantially better. The average age of the patients at the time of surgery was 66.4 years, about 3 years younger than reported for the Phase 1 and 2 implants.

The authors of the SKAR 2004 report [1] alluded to some early '… indications that the mini-incision may increase the revision rate' of UKA, and to the hazard that implants already shown to be sensitive to 'surgical routine' may experience further deterioration in their long-term results from the new operating procedure. The evidence reviewed above gives some reassurance that, in the hands of surgeons experienced in the procedure, OUKA can be performed with the same accuracy through the small incision as through the wider approach used in the past. This may be because the instruments and method of implantation of the OUKA Phase 2 implant required very little modification for use through the small incision. Indeed, the procedure is in some ways simplified by not dislocating the patella, a manoeuvre which alters the position of the femur on the tibia and makes intra-operative alignment of the components more difficult.

Education

If a specific innovation in surgery is likely to carry an increased risk of technical error during the period of learning, even for surgeons already adept in the subject in general, the case is made for a technique-specific educational course. Instructional courses for surgeons intending to perform the OUKA have been given regularly since 1998 when the Phase 3 minimally invasive technique was introduced. By the end of 2004, more than 3000 surgeons had attended. The Federal Drug Administration has recognized this as a necessity by making attendance at such a course a requirement for the practice of OUKA in the USA.

Postscript

When this chapter was already in press, the 2005 reports of the Swedish and the Australian national joint replacement registers were published [62, 63]. Table 6.9 updates Table 6.1

Table 6.9 95% confidence intervals for the risk ratio with respect to revision (SKAR 2005)

OA/UKA	n	p-value	RR	95% CI
Link–Uni	4,414		Reference	
MillerGalante	1,977	0.01	1.36	1.07–1.71
Marmor/Richards	698	0.01	1.47	1.12–1.93
Oxford	591	0.96	0.99	0.64–1.2
PFC	549	0.00	1.89	1.43–2.50
Duracon	507	0.01	1.48	1.08–2.04
Brigham	498	0.04	1.40	1.02–1.94
Genesis	403	0.45	1.20	0.75–1.90
Allegretto	258	0.13	1.37	0.91–2.08
Repicci	181	0.00	2.21	1.49–3.29
Other	58	0.94	1.08	0.15–7.72
Gender (male is ref.)		0.45	1.06	0.91–1.24
Age (per year)		0.00	0.95	0.95–0.96
Year of operation (per year)		0.62	0.99	0.95–1.03

Implants in red type had a significantly higher risk ratio than the index

(Data reproduced from the *Swedish Knee Arthroplasty Register Report 2005* with the permission of Dr O Robertsson.)

Table 6.10 Unicompartmental primary knee procedures requiring revision (AJRR 2005)[1]

Model	Number Revised	Total Number	% Revised	Observed 'component' years	Revisions per 100 observed 'component' years	Exact 95% CI
Unix	31	945	3.3	1810	1.7	(1.16, 2.43)
Repicci	41	1716	2.4	3408	1.2	(0.86, 1.63)
M/G	45	1329	3.4	2538	1.8	(1.29, 2.37)
Total	**117**	**3990**	**2.9**	**7756**	**1.5**	**(1.25, 1.81)**

Model	Number Revised	Total Number	% Revised	Observed 'component' years	Revisions per 100 observed 'component' years	Exact 95% CI
Allegretto Uni Knee	67	1238	5.4	2703	2.5	(1.92, 3.15)
Endo-Model Sled	6	310	1.9	299	2.0	(0.74, 4.37)
GRU	9	650	1.4	693	1.3	(0.59, 2.47)
Genesis	26	770	3.4	1110	2.3	(1.53, 3.43)
M/G	45	1329	3.4	2538	1,8	(1,29, 2.37)
Natural Knee	15	139	10.8	296	5,1	(2,84, 8.36)
Oxford 3	265	5471	4.8	11346	2.3	(2.06, 2.63)
PFC Sigma	9	137	6.6	476	1.9	(0.86, 3.59)
Preservation-Fixed	40	1098	4.5	1665	2.9	(2.18, 3.89)
Preservation-Mobile	33	343	9.6	584	5.7	(3.89, 7.94)
Repicci	41	1716	2.4	3408	1.2	(0.86, 1.63)
Unix	31	945	3.3	1810	1.7	(1,16, 2.43)
Others (7)	15	322	4.7	365	4,1	(2.30, 6.78)
Total	**611**	**14468**	**4.2**	**27293**	**2.2**	**(2.06, 2.42)**

Note: – Only prostheses with over 250 observed component years have been listed. The Unix, M/G and Repicci were chosen as index implants against which the other implants were compared.

(Data reproduced with permission from the *Australian Orthopaedic Association National Joint Registry Annual Report 2005*.)

and Table 6.10 updates Table 6.2. The lack of correlation in the performance of implants, within and between the registers, has persisted.

Within the SKAR, the risk of revision of two implants (Miller-Galante and Brigham) changed between 2004 and 2005 so that, of nine implants, the status of five has altered "significantly" relative to the index at least once in the four years 2002 to 2005, one of them twice (see Tables 6.8 and 6.9).

Between the SKAR and the AJRR there is no agreement. The implant with the lowest risk ratio in Sweden (OUKA) had a "significantly higher rate of revision than the comparators" in Australia; the implant with the best result in Australia (Repicci) had the worst in Sweden. The three best performing implants in Australia were chosen by the AJRR as index implants, against which others were compared, because of their low revision rates. Two of these three appear in the SKAR (Miller-Galante and Repicci) where both had significantly worse results than the index implant.

The surgeon as a variable

In the AJRR 2005 report, the revision rates of 5471 OUKA (Phase 3) were compared with those of an assemblage of 3990 UKA of three designs (Miller-Galante, Repicci and Unix) chosen as comparators because of their low revision rates. The mean revision rates of the two cohorts, 2.3 and 1.5 per 100 implant years respectively, were significantly different (Hazard Ratio 1.562; 95% CI 1.256-1.942, p<0.0001).

Although combining the results of the best three implants is a dubious statistical method, analysis of the data does demonstrate the importance of surgical expertise as the confounding variable that probably accounts for the contradictory nature of the evidence from national registers.

The AJRR made available to us the number of operations performed, and the number revised, at each of the 265 hospitals where the OUKAs were performed; and similar data for the comparator implants at 117 hospitals. To investigate the effect of patient volume, we equated hospitals that had reported fewer than 100 operations (in the 4 years that data were collected) with hospitals where a mean of less than 23 UKA per annum were performed (group A in the similar study by Robertsson et al. [14]). Since these authors had also reported decreasing failure rates with increasing throughput, we further stratified the hospitals into those that reported 100-200, 200-300 and >300. Figure 6.4 shows that the risk of revision in both cohorts was greater in hospitals with small patient volumes. For the comparator group this correlation was significant; for the OUKA it was a trend.

Fig. 6.5 shows that the two cohorts were distributed very differently among the four hospital categories. Seventy five per cent of the OUKAs were performed in hospitals reporting less than 100 operations, compared with 39 per cent of the comparators. Only 4 per cent of the OUKAs were done in a hospital reporting more than 200, compared with 34 per cent of the comparators.

Statistical analysis. Because the survival rates of both cohorts were better in large than in small surgical units, their skewed distribution among hospital categories had a profound effect on the mean revision rates of both. A statistical comparison of the two cohorts adjusted for hospital volume indicates that there was no significant difference (p=0.09) between the results. (Poisson regression analysis of the data undertaken by Dr Ly-Mee Yu, Medical Statistician, Centre for Statistics in Medicine, University of Oxford.)

Discussion

Robertsson et al. [14] found that the revision rates of the St Georg Link and the OUKA were both higher in small volume centres than in large (risk ratios 1.53 and 3.07 respectively); and the much greater dependency of the OUKA on patient volume in that study gave rise to its reputation as a "technically demanding" procedure. In the Australian data also, the revision rates of both cohorts varied inversely with the number of procedures, but it was the assemblage of fixed-bearing implants that was the more sensitive. The authors of the AJRR (2005) report wrote, referring to the study of Robertsson *et al.* [14], that they were "…unable to identify any relationship between the number of procedures performed at a hospital and the risk of revision surgery."[63]. It seems, however, that they studied only the Oxford cohort and, like us, found no more than a trend (2.5 revisions per implant year in the units performing less than 23 per annum and 2.2 in the others). Had they also studied their comparator group, they would have found a more significant effect (see Fig. 6.4).

Knutson *et al.* [64] wrote that it was "…one of the most important uses of the register to look at the cumulative revision rate of various implants, used in a large number of unselected units…" to estimate "…the outcome of the average surgery"[64]. The greatly different patterns of usage (Fig. 6.5) show that large numbers of unselected units do not ensure random distribution; and that a national register may not, therefore, measure the results of individual implants in the hands of the "average" surgeon. The outcome of the Poisson regression analysis shows how failure to account for the variable of surgical

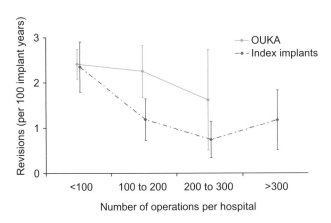

Figure 6.4 Revision rates per 100 implant years (plus 95% confidence bars) plotted against the four categories of hospitals.

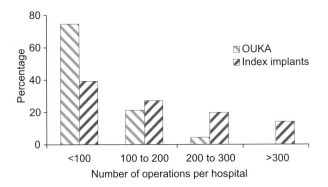

Figure 6.5 Pattern of usage. Percentages of OUKA and index implants plotted against the four categories of hospital.

experience can result in misleading conclusions. Since it was the comparator group that exhibited the greater dependence on this variable, its use for comparison with other implants in the registry may also be suspect.

Surrogate measure. The problem with attempting to adjust for surgical expertise, as is already routinely done for other variables (age and gender), is that the data on revisions in the registers is linked to hospitals and not to surgeons. Robertsson *et al.* [14] pointed out that hospital volume is only a surrogate measure and one likely to underestimate the true effect of surgical expertise, because a large patient volume in a hospital may be the work of several surgeons, and a small volume the work of one experienced practitioner. And the pattern of employment of surgeons by hospitals may differ, for instance, between Sweden and Australia [63].

One report based on an analysis of data from the New Zealand Joint Register was able to link failure rates to surgeons, not hospitals [65]. An audit of 1216 OUKA (Phase 3) performed by 73 surgeons between January 2000 and October 2003 showed a mean revision rate of 2.2 per cent. The 18 surgeons who each performed 30 or more OUKA (total 787) had a mean revision rate of 1.5%; the 33 surgeons who performed between 4 and 30 (total 391) had a revision rate of 3%; the 22 surgeons who performed three or less (total 38) had a revision rate of 8% (p=0.03; odds ratio 5.7 for comparison between high and low users).

Summary

The 2005 reports reinforce the doubts expressed earlier in this chapter on the use of national registers to compare designs of unicompartmental implant. The influence of "surgeon selection", first demonstrated by Robertsson *et al.* in Sweden, has been found to have similar force in Australia (and New Zealand), with at least as much effect on the outcome of unicompartmental arthroplasty, in both places, as implant selection. There may be differences between the sensitivity of implants to this variable but the available evidence only suggests that it is a feature of them all.

The observations imply 1) that it is at least as important to link survival data to individual surgeons as to individual designs of implant and 2) that the success of unicompartmental arthroplasty in a community will depend at least as much upon the expertise of its surgeons as upon their choice of prosthesis. The importance of implant specific instruction of surgeons needs to be emphasized.

Notes

1) Unicompartmental prostheses and their manufacturers:

Allegretto	Zimmer Inc., Warsaw, Indiana, USA
AMC Uni	Corin Group PLC, Cirencester, Gloucestershire, UK
Brigham	Johnson & Johnson, Raynham, Massachusetts, USA
Duracon	Howmedica, Rutherford, New Jersey, USA

Genesis	Smith & Nephew Richards Inc., Memphis, Tennessee, USA
Marmor	Smith & Nephew Richards Inc., Memphis, Tennessee, USA
Miller-Galante	Zimmer Inc., Warsaw, Indiana, USA
Oxford	Biomet Inc., Warsaw, Indiana, USA
PFC	Johnson & Johnson, Raynham, Massachusetts, USA
Preservation MBUKA	DePuy, Warsaw, Indiana, USA
Repicci	Biomet Inc., Warsaw, Indiana, USA
St Georg/Link Uni	Waldemar Link GmbH, Hamburg, Germany
Unix	Howmedica, Rutherford, New Jersey, USA

References

1. Lidgren L, Knutson K, Robertsson O. *Swedish Knee Arthroplasty Register: Annual Report 2004.* Lund.

2. Australian Orthopaedic Association. *National Joint Replacement Registry Annual Report.* Adelaide: 2004.

3. Murray D. Survival analysis. In: Pynsent P, Fairbank J, Carr A (ed) *Assessment Methodology in Orthopaedics.* Oxford: Butterworth-Heinemann, 1997; 19–28.

4. Murray DW, Britton AR, Bulstrode CJ. Loss to follow-up matters. *J Bone Joint Surg [Br]* 1997; **79-B**: 254–7.

5. Price AJ, Waite JC, Svard U. Long-term clinical results of the medial Oxford unicompartmental knee arthroplasty. *Clin Orthop* 2005; **435**: 171–80.

6. Emerson RH Jr, Hansborough T, Reitman RD, Rosenfeldt W, Higgins LL. Comparison of a mobile with a fixed-bearing unicompartmental knee implant. *Clin Orthop* 2002; **404**: 62–70.

7. Gleeson RE, Evans R, Ackroyd CE, Webb J, Newman JH. Fixed or mobile bearing unicompartmental knee replacement? A comparative cohort study. *Knee* 2004; **11**: 379–84.

8. Confalonieri N, Manzotti A, Pullen C. Comparison of a mobile with a fixed tibial bearing unicompartimental knee prosthesis: a prospective randomized trial using a dedicated outcome score. *Knee* 2004; **11**: 357–62.

9. Repicci JA, Eberle RW. Minimally invasive technique for unicondylar knee arthroplasty. *J South Orthop Soc* 1999; **8**: 20–7.

10. Keys GW. Reduced invasive approach for Oxford II medial unicompartmental knee replacement: a preliminary study. *Knee* 1999; **6**: 193–6.

11. Price AJ, Webb J, Topf H, Dodd CA, Goodfellow JW, Murray DW. Rapid recovery after Oxford unicompartmental arthroplasty through a short incision. *J Arthroplasty* 2001; **16**: 970–6.

12. Pandit H, Jenkins C, Barker K, Dodd CAF, Murray DW. The Oxford medial unicompartmental knee replacement using a minimally-invasive approach. *J Bone Joint Surg [Br]* 2006; **88-B**: 54–60.

13. Weale AE, Murray DW, Crawford R, Psychoyios V, Bonomo A, Howell G, O'Connor J, Goodfellow JW. Does arthritis progress in the retained compartments after 'Oxford' medial unicompartmental arthroplasty? A clinical and radiological study with a minimum ten-year follow-up. *J Bone Joint Surg [Br]* 1999; **81-B**: 783–9.

14. Robertsson O, Knutson K, Lewold S, Lidgren L. The routine of surgical management reduces failure after unicompartmental knee arthroplasty. *J Bone Joint Surg [Br]* 2001; **83-B**: 45–9.

15. Christensen NO. Unicompartmental prosthesis for gonarthrosis. A nine-year series of 575 knees from a Swedish hospital. *Clin Orthop* 1991; **273**: 165–9.

16. Grelsamer RP. Current concepts review. unicompartmental osteoarthrosis of the knee. *J Bone Joint Surg [Am]* 1995; **77-A**: 278–92.

17. Lindstrand A, Stenstrom A, Ryd L, Toksvig-Larsen S. The introduction period of unicompartmental knee arthroplasty is critical: a clinical, multicentered, and radiostereometric study of 251 Duracon unicompartmental knee arthroplasties. *J Arthroplasty* 2000; **15**: 608–16.

18. Jeer PJ, Keene GC, Gill P. Unicompartmental knee arthroplasty: an intermediate report of survivorship after the introduction of a new system with analysis of failures. *Knee* 2004; **11**: 369–74.

19. Rees JL, Price AJ, Beard DJ, Dodd CA, Murray DW. Minimally invasive Oxford unicompartmental knee arthroplasty: functional results at 1 year and the effect of surgical inexperience. *Knee* 2004; **11**: 363–7.

20. Keys GW, Ul-Abiddin Z, Toh EM. Analysis of first forty Oxford medial unicompartmental knee replacement from a small district hospital in UK. *Knee* 2004; **11**: 375–7.

21. Lewold S, Goodman S, Knutson K, Robertsson O, Lidgren L. Oxford meniscal bearing knee versus the Marmor knee in unicompartmental arthroplasty for arthrosis. A Swedish multicenter survival study. *J Arthroplasty* 1995; **10**: 722–31.

22. Svard UC, Price AJ. Oxford medial unicompartmental knee arthroplasty. A survival analysis of an independent series. *J Bone Joint Surg [Br]* 2001; **83-B**: 191–4.

23. Price AJ. Medial meniscal bearing unicompartmental arthroplasty: wear, mechanics and clinical outcome. DPhil Thesis, University of Oxford, 2003.

24. Marmor L. Unicompartmental arthroplasty of the knee with a minimum ten-year follow-up period. *Clin Orthop* 1988; **228**: 171–7.

25. Witvoet J, Peyrache MD, Nizard R. Protheses unicompartimentaire du genou type 'Lotus' dans le traitement des gonarthroses lateralisées. *Rev Chirurg Orthop* 1993; **7**: 565–76.

26. Knutson K, Lewold S, Robertsson O, Lidgren L. The Swedish Knee Arthroplasty Register. a nation-wide study of 30 003 knees 1976–1992. *Acta Orthop Scand* 1994; **65**: 375–86.

27. Devereaux PJ, Bhandari M, Clarke M, Montori VM, Cook DJ, Yusuf S, Sackett DL, Cina CS, Walter SD, Haynes B, Schunemann HJ, Norman GR, Guyatt GH. Need for expertise based randomised controlled trials. *BMJ* 2005; **330**(7482): 88.

28. Kozinn SC, Scott R. Unicondylar knee arthroplasty. *J Bone Joint Surg [Am]* 1989; **71-A**: 145–50.

29. Stern SH, Becker MW, Insall JN. Unicondylar knee arthroplasty. An evaluation of selection criteria. *Clin Orthop* 1993; **286**: 143–8.

30. Ritter MA, Faris PM, Thong AE, Davis KE, Meding JB, Berend ME. Intra-operative findings in varus osteoarthritis of the knee. An analysis of pre-operative alignment in potential candidates for unicompartmental arthroplasty. *J Bone Joint Surg [Br]* 2004; **86-B**: 43–7.

31. Berger RA, Meneghini RM, Jacobs JJ, Sheinkop MB, DellaValle CT, Rosenberg AG, Galante JO Results of unicompartmental knee arthroplasty at a minimum of ten years of follow-up. *J Bone Joint Surg [Am]* 2005; **87-A**: 999–1006.

32. Capra SW, Fehring TK. Unicondylar arthroplasty. A survivorship analysis. *J Arthroplasty* 1992; **7** 247–51.

33. Heck DA, Marmor L, Gibson A, Rougraff BT. Unicompartmental knee arthroplasty. A multicenter investigation with long-term follow-up evaluation. *Clin Orthop* 1993; **286**: 154–9.

34. Cartier P, Sanouiller JL, Grelsamer RP. Unicompartmental knee arthroplasty surgery. 10-year minimum follow-up period. *J Arthroplasty* 1996; **11**: 782–8.

35. Tabor OB, Jr., Tabor OB. Unicompartmental arthroplasty: a long-term follow-up study. *Arthroplasty* 1998: **13**: 373–9.

36. Squire MW, Callaghan JJ, Goetz DD, Sullivan PM, Johnston RC. Unicompartmental knee replacement. A minimum 15 year follow up study. *Clin Orthop* 1999; **367**: 61–72.

37. Neider E. Schlitten prothese, Rotations knie and Scharnierprothese modell St. Georg and Endo-Modell. *Orthopade* 1991; **20**: 170–180.

38. Weale AE, Newman JH. Unicompartmental arthroplasty and high tibial osteotomy for osteoarthrosis of the knee. A comparative study with a 12- to 17-year follow-up period. *Clin Orthop* 1994; **302**: 134–7.

39. Ansari S, Newman JH, Ackryd CE. St. Georg sledge for medial compartmental knee replacement. 461 arthroplasties followed for 4 (1–17) years. *Acta Orthop Scand* 1997; **68**: 430–4.

40. Scott RD, Cobb AG, McQueary FG, Thornhill TS. Unicompartmental knee arthroplasty. Eight- to 12-year follow-up evaluation with survivorship analysis. *Clin Orthop* 1999; **271**: 96–100.

41. Hasegawa Y, Ooishi Y, Shimizu T, Sugiura H, Takahashi S, Ito H, Iwata H. Unicompartmental knee arthroplasty for medial gonarthrosis: 5 to 9 years follow-up evaluation of 77 knees. *Arch Orthop Trauma Surg* 1998; **117**: 183–7.

42. Bert JM. 10-year survivorship of metal-backed, unicompartmental arthroplasty. *J Arthroplasty* 1998; **13**: 901–5.

43. Berger RA, Nedeff DD, Barden RM, Sheinkop MM, Jacobs JJ, Rosenberg AG, Galante JO. Unicompartmental knee arthroplasty. Clinical experience at 6- 10-year followup. *Clin Orthop* 1999; **367**: 50–60.

44. Argenson JN, Chevrol-Benkeddache Y, Aubaniac JM. Modern unicompartmental knee arthroplasty with cement: a three to ten-year follow-up study. *J Bone Joint Surg [Am]* 2002; **84-A**: 2235–9.

45. Ritter MA, Berend ME, Meding JB, Keating EM, Faris PM, Crites BM. Long-term followup of anatomic graduated components posterior cruciate-retaining total knee replacement. *Clin Orthop* 2001; **388**: 51–7.

46. Robertsson O, Scott G, Freeman MA. Ten-year survival of the cemented Freeman-Samuelson primary knee arthroplasty. Data from the Swedish Knee Arthroplasty Register and the Royal London Hospital. *J Bone Joint Surg [Br]* 2000; **82-B**: 506–7.

47. Laskin RS. The Genesis total knee prosthesis. *Clin Orthop* 2001; **388**: 95–102.

48. Brassard MF, Insall JN, Scuderi GR, Colizza W. Does modularity affect clinical success? A comparison with a minimum 10-year follow up. *Clin Orthop* 2001; **388**: 26–32.

49. Malkani AL, Rand JA, Bryan RS, Wallrichs SL. Total knee arthroplasty with the kinematic condylar prosthesis. A ten-year follow-up study. *J Bone Joint Surg [Am]* 1995; **77-A**: 423–31.

50. Weir DJ, Moran CG, Pinder IM. Kinematic condylar total knee arthroplasty. 14-year survivorship analysis of 208 consecutive cases. *J Bone Joint Surg [Br]* 1996; **78-B**: 907–11.

51. Berger RA, Lyon JH, Jacobs JJ, Barden RM, Barkson EM, Sheinkop MB, Rosenberg AG, Galante JO Problems with cementless total knee arthroplasty at 11 years follow up. *Clin Orthop* 2001; **392**: 196–207.

52. Berger RA, Rosenberg AG, Barden RM, Sheinkop MB, Jacobs JJ, Galante JO. Long term follow-up of the Miller–Galante total knee replacement. *Clin Orthop* 2001; **388**: 58–67.

53. Colizza WA, Insall JN, Scuderi GR. The posterior stabilized total knee prosthesis. Assessment of polyethylene damage and osteolysis after a ten-year-minimum follow-up. *J Bone Joint Surg [Am]* 1995; **77-A**: 1713–20.

54. Ranawat C, Flynn WF, Saddler S, Hansraj KK, Maynard MJ. Long term results of the total condylar knee arthroplasty. *Clin Orthop* 1993; **286**: 94–102.

55. Pavone V, Boettner F, Fickert S, Sculco TP. Total condylar knee arthroplasty: a long-term follow up. *Clin Orthop* 2001; **388**: 18–25.

56. Gill GS, Joshi AB, Mills DM. Total condylar knee arthroplasty. 16- to 21-year results. *Clin Orthop* 1999; **367**: 210–15.

57. Rodriguez JA, Brende H, Ranawat C. Total condylar knee replacement. *Clin Orthop* 2001; **388**: 10–17.

58. Kumar A, Fiddian NJ. Medial compartment arthroplasty of the knee. *Knee* 1999; **6**: 21–3.

59. Murray DW, Goodfellow JW, O'Connor JJ. The Oxford medial unicompartmental arthroplasty: a ten-year survival study. *J Bone Joint Surg [Br]* 1998; **80-B**: 983–9.

60. Rajasekhar C, Das S, Smith A. Unicompartmental knee arthroplasty. 2- to 12-year results in a community hospital. *J Bone Joint Surg [Br]* 2004; **86-B**: 983–5.

61. Vorlat P, Van Isacker T, Pouliart N, Handebrug F, Casteleyn PP, Gheysen F, Verdonk R. *Knee Surg Sports Traumatol Arthrosc* 2006; **14**: 40–5.

62. Lidgren L, Knutson K, Robertsson O. *Swedish Knee Arthroplasty Register: Annual Report 2005*; Lund.

63. Australian Orthopaedic Association. *National Joint Replacement Registry Annual Report*, Adelaide; ANJR, 2005

64. Knutson K, Lewold S, Robertsson O, Lidgren L. The Swedish knee arthroplasty register. *Acta Orthop Scand* 1994; **65**: 375–386.

65. Hartnett N, Hobbs A, Rothwell A, Tregonning R. *The early failure of the Oxford Phase 3 unicompartmental arthroplasty*. Presented at the Annual Meeting of the New Zealand Orthopaedic Association. October 4th 2005; Christchurch: New Zealand.

7

Management of complications

Sources

In this chapter we describe how failures occur in UKA in general, and OUKA in particular, and suggest ways of dealing with them. We also suggest some common causes of failure and how errors can be avoided.

The clinical content of the text is based on the first-hand experience of the authors and on numerous second-hand reports received from colleagues seeking advice on management or reporting their experiences at OUKA user-group meetings. Since our practical experience is exclusively with the meniscal bearing implant, data on fixed-bearing implants has been taken from the literature, mainly the SKAR reports. These provide the distribution, in percentages, of the causes for revision of UKA from the accumulated data of all the implants used in the last decade, the great majority of which were fixed-bearing designs. Unfortunately, the causes of failure are given in rather broad categories; for instance 'loosening' does not specify which component is affected, nor does 'progression' say whether the arthritis has extended to the patellofemoral or to the contralateral compartment. The only source of information from SKAR specific to OUKA is that given by Lewold *et al.* [1] who described the causes for revision of 50 failed Oxford implants (Phases 1 and 2) in 699 knees collected from the SKAR database between 1983 and 1992.

Complications occur more commonly in the hands of learners than in those of the experienced surgeons whose reports are published in the literature, and so statistical conclusions drawn from cohort studies are necessarily biased.

Infection

The SKAR 2004 report [2] showed a lower risk of revision for infection in UKA than in TKA. The authors commented that '... although the UKA has been shown to have a substantially higher CRR than the TKA, the number of serious complications such as infection/arthrodesis/amputation is much less'. In the study by Lewold *et al.* [1], the frequency of revision for infection in OUKA was 0.6 per cent. In the OUKA Phase 3 cohort implanted through a small incision, the frequency of revision for infection was also 0.6 per cent.

Diagnosis

The methods of investigation of suspected infection are the same in OUKA as in TKA except that radionuclide uptake studies are not helpful. After OUKA, activity in the bone beneath the implants persists for several years, and so the presence of a 'hot' area on the scan is not necessarily evidence of infection (or loosening). The C-reactive protein or erythrocyte sedimentation rate are the most useful diagnostic tests but may not be positive in the first 2–3 weeks.

Treatment

Acute infection

In the immediate postoperative period, acute infection is diagnosed and treated in the same way as after TKA. Early open debridement and intravenous antibodies can arrest the infection and save the arthroplasty.

Late infection

Failure of treatment of an acute infection, or infection of later onset, is diagnosed from the clinical and radiological signs and bacteriological studies, as in TKA. The earliest radiological signs may be in the retained compartment. Figure 7.1(a) shows thinning of the articular cartilage and porosis at the joint margins in the lateral compartment of an infected knee after medial OUKA; evidence of chondrolysis by the infecting organism and chronic synovitis. (Note that acute rheumatoid synovitis can produce a similar appearance.) The eventual appearance of thick (<2 mm) ill-defined radiolucencies beneath the components (Fig. 7.1(b)), quite different from the thin radiolucent lines with radiodense margins that outline most normally functioning OUKA, is diagnostic.

Treatment is by removal of the implant and excision of the inflammatory membrane, followed by one- or two-stage revision to TKA. We prefer the two-stage procedure, with removal of the implant and excision of the articular surfaces of the retained compartment at the first stage. An antibiotic-loaded spacer is left in the joint to maintain the gap and allow movement until the infection is eradicated and the second stage can be safely undertaken. Three types of spacer can be used (Fig. 7.2). We favour a bicompartmental spacer as this allows removal of all infected articular cartilage at the first stage. The second-stage TKA usually requires a stemmed tibial implant as there is often substantial tibial bone loss.

Medial tibial plateau fracture

'Fracture' (type unspecified) constituted about 1 per cent of the reasons for revision of UKA reported by SKAR in the decade 1992–2001 [2]. No fracture was reported either by Lewold et al. [1] in 699 OUKAs nor by Pandit et al. in 688 OUKA Phase 3 [3]. Four plateau fractures occurred in 62 UKAs reported by Berger et al. [4] and there are other occasional reports in the literature [5–7].

Despite the very few fractures in the published reports of OUKA cohorts, several have been reported to us by other users and we believe that the complication is more common than the literature suggests, particularly among surgeons beginning to do unicompartmental arthroplasty and in populations with constitutionally small tibias (e.g. Asian populations).

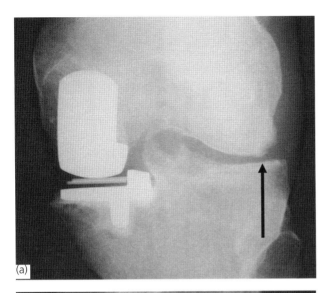

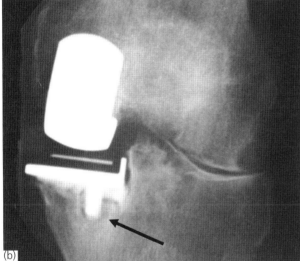

Figure 7.1 (a) The earliest radiographic sign of infection may be the appearance of subchondral erosions in the retained compartment of the knee. (b) The radiolucencies under the tibial plateau are more than 1 mm thick and are not defined by a radiodense line. They are different from the common 'physiological' radiolucent lines and suggest infection and/or loosening.

Causes

It seems likely that most, if not all, plateau fractures occur intraoperatively although they are often not diagnosed until later, commonly at 2–12 weeks (Fig. 7.3(a)). If the fracture is initially undisplaced, it may not be visible on the immediate postoperative radiographs, only appearing later when weight-bearing has caused displacement, and postoperative pain and deformity have drawn attention to the problem.

Weakening of the condyle

Weakening of the condyle by removal of its articular surface is probably the main reason for fracture. Since this is unavoidable, great care is taken to avoid any additional

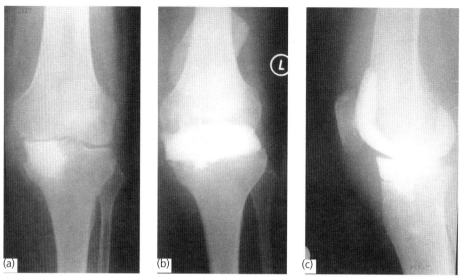

Figure 7.2 Spacers are used between the procedures of a two-stage revision for infection:
(a) unicompartmental (not recommended as bacteria can persist in retained cartilage);
(b) simple bicompartmental; (c) articulating.

weakening of the bone. We believe that the most potent cause of fracture is damage to the posterior cortex and the cancellous bone by vertical saw cuts that go deeper than they need (Fig. 7.3(b)). These weaken the bone about as much as excising an additional 20 mm layer of bone. Even the two small holes made in the anterior cortex by the nails that fix the tibial saw guide have been shown to decrease the strength of the condyle [5,7]. However, we have used this method of fixation in all phases of the OUKA without complication and do not believe that it is the cause of fracture.

The more bone that is removed from the condyle, the weaker is the remainder; therefore the surgical objective should be to remove as little as possible. It is an advantage of meniscal-bearing arthroplasty that polyethylene only 4 mm thick can be used safely. This advantage should be exploited by removing as little tibial plateau as possible.

The smaller the tibia, the less bone can be safely removed from it. This may explain why more fractures have been reported to us from countries where many adults are of small stature (Japan, Korea). Extra-small implants should be used in such patients and we recommend that, in them, the horizontal tibial saw cut should aim to accommodate a thin bearing which can be as little as 3 mm thick (see Chapter 3).

Application of excessive force

Application of excessive force is the other factor in causing fracture. The heavy hammer commonly used in TKA is not appropriate for UKA. A small hammer, in the hands of a surgeon alert to the risk, will seldom cause a tibial plateau fracture.

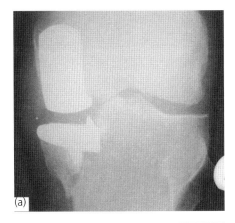

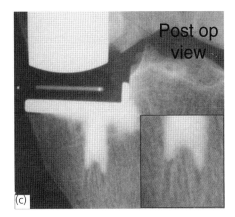

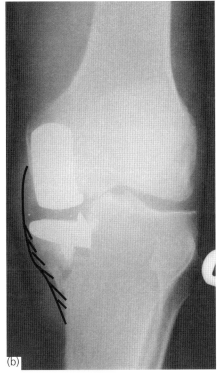

Figure 7.3 (a) Displaced fracture of the medial tibial condyle. (b) The bearing does not dislocate because the width of the 'gap' is maintained by the intact MCL. (c) The probable cause of fracture is the deep vertical saw cuts made during preparation of the groove for the tibial keel. In this case, the cuts (seen here as radiolucent) are about twice the depth of the tibial keel.

Pathological anatomy

Figure 7.3(b) shows how the strong attachments of the MCL to the cortex of the medial tibial plateau maintain the components of the arthroplasty in their proper relationship. In particular, the gap between the femoral and tibial implants remains unaltered, and dislocation of the bearing does not occur. Displacement of the fragment distally allows the tibiofemoral axis to drift into varus.

Treatment

Management depends on the stage at which the fracture is diagnosed and the degree of varus deformity.

Intraoperative diagnosis

Several reports suggest that if the fracture is diagnosed during the operation it should be reduced and internally fixed. Thereafter, the UKA can be completed in the expectation of a good result [8].

Postoperative diagnosis

The following algorithm is suggested.

Within 12 weeks of surgery:

A If the fracture is minimally displaced, or undisplaced employ external splinting to maintain alignment while awaiting union.

B If there is significant displacement, employ open reduction and internal fixation with an AO buttress plate or interfragmentary screws.

Later than 12 weeks after surgery:

A If the fracture is united and not unacceptably displaced, no action is required.

B If the fracture is united but causing pain, suspect tibial component loosening. If this is confirmed revise to a TKA.

C If the fracture is not united, revise to a TKA with a stemmed tibial component. (Mobilise the fragment and freshen its edges, use bone graft from the lateral compartment, reduce and fix with an AO plate or interfragmentary screws.)

What constitutes 'acceptable' varus deformity? In this context, up to 5° of varus is probably acceptable. In UKA, varus malalignment does not have the same sinister implication as it has in TKA; indeed, many practitioners aim always to leave the operated limb in a few degrees of varus.

Dislocation of a mobile bearing

This complication was introduced into surgery with the invention of mobile-bearing knee arthroplasty [9]. SKAR reports do not include it in their list of complications, but Lewold *et al.* [1], using SKAR data, found that the risk was 2.3 per cent and that it was the most common cause of failure in OUKA Phase 1 and 2 (16 out of 50 revisions). Most of these dislocations occurred early: 10 in the first year and four in the second (mean 17 months). Price [10] found a difference in the rates of dislocation between OUKA Phase 1 (2.5 per cent) and Phase 2 (0.5 per cent). In the Phase 3 cohort [3] it was 0.2 per cent. Jeer *et al.* [11] described a consecutive series of 66 LCS mobile-bearing UKAs followed for a mean of 5.9 years (range 5.1–6.6) with no instance of dislocation of a bearing.

Causes

Primary dislocations, due to inadequate entrapment of the bearing, are the most common. They occur early and are due to surgical error.

The following mistakes all diminish the bearing's entrapment (the mechanism of entrapment is explained in detail in Chapter 3).

1. Inequality of the 90° and 20° flexion gaps.
2. Femoral component (and therefore the bearing) sited too far from the lateral wall of the tibial component, so that the bearing is free to rotate through 90°.
3. Intraoperative damage to the MCL (or ACL).
4. Failure to remove osteophytes from the back of the femoral condyle causing impingement in flexion and anterior displacement of the bearing, particularly in patients who achieve high degrees of flexion.
5. Cement protruding above the tibial plateau surface.
6. A bearing that is too thin relative to gap width may, theoretically, dislocate, and beginners, fearful of dislocation, tend to insert the thickest bearing possible, but this is a mistake. 'Overstuffing' the knee should be avoided as it causes other problems.

Secondary dislocation is the result of loss of entrapment from loosening (and subsidence) of the metal components. Spontaneous elongation of ligaments over time does not seem to occur unless there is impingement, when forced flexion or extension may stretch ligaments.

Traumatic dislocation has occasionally been encountered when a normally functioning OUKA has been forced into an extreme posture and the MCL has been momentarily stretched.

Diagnosis

Dislocation occurs when the knee is unloaded or at the moment when load is re-applied, for example rising from a chair or getting out of bed. It is usually a dramatic event and the patient seeks urgent advice, but dislocation can occur relatively silently. Walking may be resumed with the bearing displaced; the weight is borne (painlessly) through the opposed metal components.

Radiographs demonstrate the site of the displaced bearing, and may suggest its cause (e.g. osteophytes, retained cement, or displacement of a metal component).

Since the anterior rim of the bearing is higher than its posterior rim, posterior dislocation requires more distraction of the joint than anterior dislocation. Therefore the displaced bearing is most commonly found in the anterior joint space, often in the suprapatellar pouch (Fig. 7.4(a)). Displacement into the posterior joint space (Fig. 7.4(b)) suggests that the bearing has rotated through 90° (point (2) above), from which position it is as easy for it to dislocate backwards as forwards. Occasionally, the bearing is found to be tilted into the intercondylar space where it may stabilize in a subluxed position (see section on lateral compartment osteoarthritis in Chapter 2).

Treatment

Manipulation can result in relocation. On a few occasions reduction has occurred, more or less spontaneously, under anaesthesia. However, **arthrotomy** is almost always required to remove the bearing and to determine the cause of its displacement. The bearing can

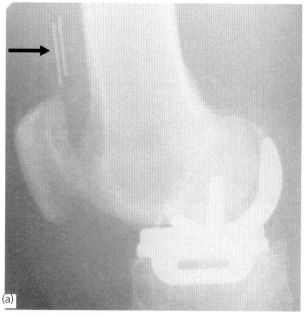

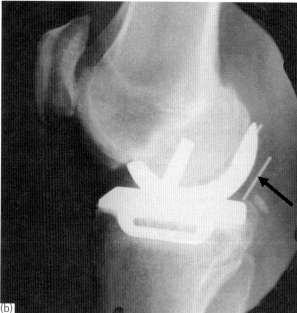

Figure 7.4 (a) Anterior and (b) posterior dislocation of the bearing.

usually be retrieved through a small anterior incision, even if it is in the back of the joint, but an additional posterior arthrotomy has sometimes been needed. The femoral component was dislodged on one occasion while retrieving the bearing and was successfully re-cemented.

Primary dislocation

When both the metal components are found to be securely fixed to the bones, other causes of dislocation need to be sought.

Any bone or cement that might impinge on the bearing is removed and an anatomical bearing is inserted (see Chapter 3). It is important not to over tighten the ligaments.

If there is recurrent dislocation, MCL damage or a serious mismatch between the 90° and 20° flexion gaps, TKA should be performed.

Since the introduction of a fixed-bearing tibial plateau to articulate with the OUKA femoral component some surgeons have converted to this in cases where instability of the mobile bearing is the only defect in the arthroplasty. However, it should be noted that SKAR data demonstrate that revisions of failed UKA to another UKA have generally been less successful than revisions from UKA to TKA.

Secondary dislocation

This is dealt with in the section below on loosening of a fixed component.

Traumatic dislocation

The few patients in which this has occurred have been successfully managed by either closed reduction of the displaced bearing or open insertion of a new bearing.

Loosening of a fixed component

In the SKAR 2004 report [2], the most common cause for failure of UKA was loosening of a component. About 50 per cent of revisions were for this cause (cf. about 30 per cent of TKA revisions). Lewold *et al.* [1] found that the risk of revision of OUKA for loosening was 2.1 per cent. It was the second most common cause of failure (28 per cent). Many components loosened early; the mean time to revision from this cause was 26 months (range 6–74 months). So far, there have been no revisions for loosening in the 688 Phase 3 implants followed for up to 7 years [3].

Diagnosis

In OUKA, the only reliable radiographic evidence for loosening of a metal component is its displacement. For example, a loose tibial component may tilt or a femoral component rotate about is peg. As has been discussed elsewhere, stable radiolucencies are very common at the bone–cement interfaces and are not evidence of loosening. Displacement is diagnosed by comparing two radiographs taken with a time interval between them; however, small changes in position can only be detected if the X-ray beam was aligned, on both occasions, in the same relation to one of the components. The required accuracy can only be achieved if both radiographs were taken with the beam aligned by fluoroscopy (Fig. 7.5).

Misinterpretation of the 'physiological' lucencies so commonly seen on fluoroscopically aligned radiographs has resulted in unnecessary revision by surgeons unfamiliar with their benign nature.

Occasionally, dislocation of the bearing draws attention to a loose component.

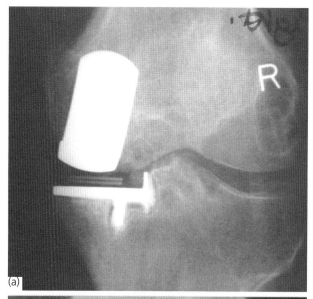

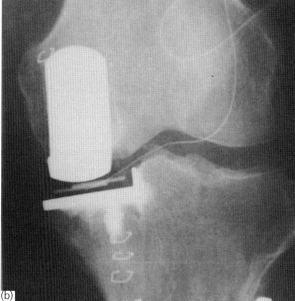

Figure 7.5 (a) This (fluoroscopically aligned) radiograph was misinterpreted as evidence of loosening of the tibial component. However, the radiolucencies beneath that component are thin and defined by a radiodense line, suggesting that they are stable and benign. When this radiograph is compared with (b) the (similarly fluoroscopically aligned) radiograph, taken immediately postoperatively, the late displacement of the femoral component is obvious. At the revision operation, the tibial component was found to be firmly fixed and the femoral component was loose.

Causes

Early failures are probably the result of poor initial fixation. Immediate postoperative radiographs and retrieved specimens have often revealed unsatisfactory cementing of the tibial component, and we have had several reports of sudden displacement of the femoral component in the immediate postoperative period, attributable (in retrospect) to poor initial fixation of its posterior facet. Some evidence from the retrieval studies suggests that late failures may be due to the accumulated effects of impact loading from impingement of the front of the bearing on the femoral condyle in full extension.

Treatment

In **early loosening**, if the bone socket has not been seriously eroded, re-cementing the component is a reasonable option and has been successful on several occasions.

However, in **late loosening**, the bone will already be more extensively damaged and revision to TKA is better undertaken immediately.

Lateral compartment arthritis

In the SKAR 2004 report [2], about 25 per cent of UKA revisions were for 'progression' of arthritis, but whether in the patellofemoral or the contralateral compartment was not specified.

Lewold *et al.* [1] found a rate of revision of OUKA for contralateral arthrosis of 1.4 per cent, accounting for 20 per cent of all revisions. The mean time for revision from this cause was 21 months (range 5–48 months).

Diagnosis

Pain in the knee, usually but not always on the lateral side, is the main symptom. The first radiographic sign is narrowing of the lateral compartment joint space (Fig. 7.6), and this may long precede the onset of pain. Subchondral sclerosis and disappearance of the joint space ensue. Osteophytes around the margins of the lateral compartment are very common and do not necessarily portend progressive arthritis.

Causes

Some authors have regarded arthritis of the contralateral compartment in UKA as a time-dependent consequence of the gradual spread of osteoarthritis throughout the joint [12], perhaps hastened by the presence within the joint cavity of the foreign materials of the prosthesis. If this were true, presumably the incidence of failure from this cause would rise steadily with the passage of time, but there is some evidence that lateral arthritis causes short- and mid-term failure. Thus it was the most common cause of revision in the 439 OUKA reviewed by Price *et al.* [13] but was not reported after the eighth year, although there were 139 knees at risk at 10 years and 26 at 15 years.

Most authors believe, as we do, that overcorrection of the varus deformity into valgus (Fig. 7.7) is the usual cause, and many surgeons recommend aiming to leave the UKA knee in a few degrees of varus to avoid this. Choosing the postoperative tibiofemoral angle is not an option in the OUKA operation since the thickness of the bearing is selected to match the lengths of the ligaments, not to provide an arbitrary alignment of the limb. Therefore an intact MCL is all-important if overcorrection is to be avoided. The tibial saw guide used in the Phase 2 OUKA had a medial extension which lay along the medial side of the tibia close to the MCL (Fig. 7.8), and its insertion required detachment of some of the deepest fibres of the ligament from the bone. In the Phase 1 procedures,

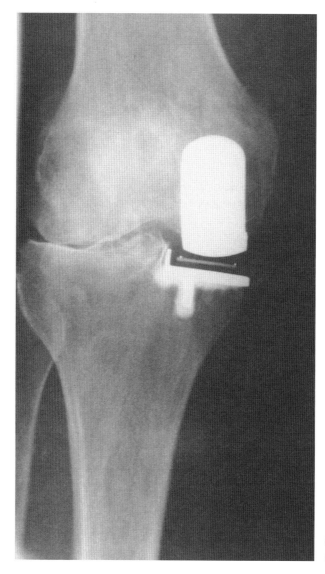

Figure 7.6 Severe lateral compartment degeneration.

the saw guide was applied only to the anterior surface of the tibia and no fibres of the MCL needed to be detached. This difference in technique may explain the finding that lateral compartment arthritis accounted for about half the failures in Phase 2 implants and none of the failures in Phase 1 implants [10].

In 688 Phase 3 implants (followed for 1–7 years), no knee has yet failed from lateral compartment arthritis. The Phase 3 tibial saw guide is similar to the one used with the Phase 1 implant, so perhaps the risk of lateral compartment arthritis will be less than in the Phase 2 implant. However, some radiographic evidence of progress of lateral arthritis was found in 5 of the 101 knees followed for 5+ years.

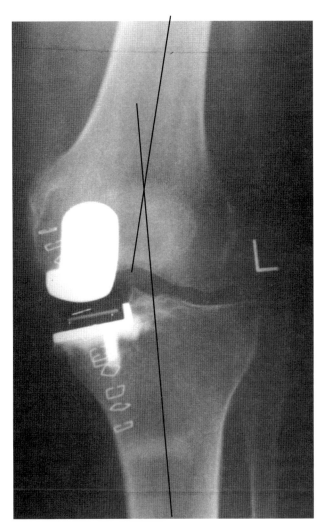

Figure 7.7 Postoperative radiograph of a knee overcorrected into valgus. Such a degree of valgus could only occur after damage to the MCL.

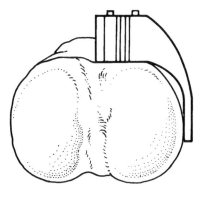

Figure 7.8 Plan view of the OUKA (Phase 2) tibial saw guide (see text).

We recommend very careful intraoperative preservation of the MCL (particularly its deep fibres) and avoidance of 'overstuffing' of the medial compartment with a thicker bearing than the ligaments will easily accommodate.

Treatment

If the symptoms warrant surgical treatment, revision to TKA is indicated.

Persistent unexplained pain

In the SKAR reports there is no category for 'pain' as a cause for revision of UCA. Only two of the 50 OUKA revisions reported by Lewold *et al.* [1] (4 months and 21 months) were for pain. However, unexplained persistent pain has appeared in cohort studies as a cause for revision of unicompartmental replacements.

Causes

Pain is most commonly felt anteromedially but can occur at any site around the knee. Possible explanations include tibial condyle overload, overhang of the tibial component, overstretching of the MCL (bearing too thick) and pes anserinus bursitis. 'Overloading' of the cortices of the tibial condyle was demonstrated by strain gauges when the OUKA tibial component was loaded in cadavers in the laboratory, and it probably occurs after every procedure. Therefore it does not readily explain the pain felt by a few patients.

Diagnosis

From some cases in our own practice, and from numerous reports at OUKA user-group meetings, we have come to recognize a pattern of symptoms as follows:

The site of the pain is nearly always anteromedial, at or below the level of the joint line. Its onset is commonly a few weeks to a few months after the operation. It is sometimes felt from the day of surgery and rarely starts more than 6 months after the operation. The pain is moderate to severe; it is sometimes continuous but made worse by weight-bearing.

Physical examination reveals no consistent associated signs except local tenderness to palpation at the medial joint line or close to it. Joint effusion is commonly found in the first months after surgery but is not more common in painful knees. The range of movement is usually good and the joint functions well, usually with a normal gait despite the pain.

Referred pain from hip or lumbar spinal disease must always be excluded.

Radiographs of the knee are normal. However, the physiological radiolucent line beneath the tibial plateau begins to appear at 6–12 months, and its presence in a knee that is painful may easily be misinterpreted as evidence of tibial component loosening. Revision to TKA in these circumstances is not only unnecessary but is often ineffective in relieving the pain. As has been mentioned above, the only reliable radiographic sign of loosening of a component is its displacement (relative to the other component) in sequential fluoroscopically aligned radiographs.

We have not found radionuclide bone scans useful for the assessment of pain as 'hot' scans are frequently found in well-functioning OUKAs many years after the index procedure.

MRI scanning has occasionally been useful. For example, it can demonstrate a lateral meniscal tear with lateral pain. A normal MRI in association with a normal radiograph can provide useful reassurance for a patient who is, correctly, being treated conservatively in the expectation that the pain will settle spontaneously.

Arthroscopy is occasionally used for the investigation of pain. Of course, patellofemoral joint degeneration is often seen (see Chapter 2), but there is no evidence of its association with pain and we do not believe that its presence justifies revision. Arthroscopy is particularly useful in detecting femoral component loosening.

Persistent pain sometimes follows use of the OUKA for the wrong indications. We have encountered persistent pain in several knees in which the surgeon failed to demonstrate full-thickness cartilage loss in the medial compartment on the preoperative radiographs or eburnated bone at arthroscopy. Our indications for OUKA do *not* include moderate, or even severe, surface degeneration of the cartilage surfaces as seen by arthroscopy. Full-thickness cartilage loss from both surfaces of the medial compartment and the presence of eburnated bone are the circumstances that cause severe pain and, in our view, justify joint replacement. If partial-thickness loss seldom causes pain, UKA for that indication will not reliably relieve the pain.

Natural history

The natural history of this syndrome is benign. In all but a few cases, the pain resolves in time, usually by the second year.

Treatment

After appropriate investigations have revealed no cause, the patient needs to be reassured that the prognosis is good. We have found several treatments to be useful in controlling the pain, including injections of local anaesthetic and cortisone, anti-inflammatory drugs, splinting the knee, and decreasing the patient's activities.

There are isolated reports of cure by excision of a neuroma, injection of the pes ansarinus bursa, and downsizing the bearing (on the supposition that the pain is due to excess tension in the MCL) or converting it to an anatomic bearing. We have little personal experience of these interventions and generally advise against further surgery.

The patient with pain that persists after UKA is at risk from the bias towards early revision to TKA referred to in Chapter 6. No arthroplasty cures the pain in every case, and the 5–6 per cent of 'unsatisfied' patients discovered in the SKAR 2004 survey of knee arthroplasties [2] must have included some with unexplained pain. Those with pain after UKA may be offered TKA, as the next therapeutic step, more readily than those who already have a TKA. Psychoyios *et al.* [14] traced four of six patients who had been treated by TKA for unexplained pain after OUKA and found that in three of them the pain persisted. Such procedures are often not only unnecessary but also ineffective.

We have found that the patient's fears can often be allayed, and an unnecessary revision usually avoided, by referral to another surgeon experienced in UKA for a second opinion.

Recurrent haemarthrosis

This is a rare complication of OUKA, as it is of TKA. The haemarthroses are usually of sudden onset and sometimes acute enough to demand aspiration for relief of pain. Each episode is usually short-lived, interfering with function for a few days, and subsiding spontaneously, but recurring, often several times.

Cause

The probable cause is recurrent mechanical damage to hypertrophic synovium.

Management

If a blood-clotting disorder is excluded, the prognosis for spontaneous cessation of the episodes is good. However, one of the few patients with this complication in our practice continued to bleed intermittently for some months until he was cured by a limited excision of hypertrophic synovium.

Limited motion

Knee movements are usually recovered rapidly, particularly since we have used a small incision without dislocation of the patella. Early flexion need not be encouraged since it occurs spontaneously in most patients. Occasionally, however, manipulation under anaesthesia has been employed if the knee has not recovered 90° flexion at 6 weeks. In these cases, unlike manipulation of a stiff joint after TKA, there are no adhesions in the suprapatellar pouch that need to be ruptured and the knee flexes fully with the application of little force.

Extension improves spontaneously after OUKA and seldom lacks more than 1°–2° at the end of the first year.

Fracture of the bearing

Three instances of fracture of an OUKA bearing have been reported in the literature [13,15]. Two bearings fractured after trauma and one apparently spontaneously. We have also been told about a few other fractures. When the thickness of the bearing was known, it was always the thinnest (3.5 mm). Treatment is by replacement with a new bearing.

We now advise against implanting the thinnest bearing except in small patients (usually women) for whom the small or extra-small femoral components are used. In those cases the risk of intraoperative fracture, from removal of more tibial bone, may be greater than the risk of fracture of the thin bearing.

Patellofemoral osteoarthritis

Patellofemoral arthritis was discussed in Chapter 2.

References

1. Lewold S, Goodman S, Knutson K, Robertsson O, Lidgren L. Oxford meniscal bearing knee versus the Marmor knee in unicompartmental arthroplasty for arthrosis. A Swedish multicenter survival study. *J Arthroplasty* 1995; **10**: 722–31.

2. Lidgren L, Knutson K, Robertsson O. *Swedish Knee Arthroplasty Register: Annual Report 2004.* Lund: Swedish Knee Arthroplasty Register, 2004.

3. Pandit H, Jenkins C, Barker K, Dodd CAF, Murray DW. The Oxford medial unicompartmental knee replacement using a minimally invasive approach. *J Bone Joint Surg [Br]* 2006; **88-B**: 54–60.

4. Berger RA, Nedeff DD, Barden RM, Sheinkop MM, Jacobs JJ, Rosenberg AG, Galante JO. Unicompartmental knee arthroplasty. Clinical experience at 6- to 10-year follow-up. *Clin Orthop* 1999; **367**: 50–60.

5. Swanson AB, Swanson GD, Powers T, Khalil MA, Maupin BK, Mayhew DE, Moss SH. Unicompartmental and bicompartmental arthroplasty of the knee with a finned metal tibial-plateau implant. *J Bone Joint Surg [Am]* 1985; **67-A**: 1175–82.

6. Yang KY, Yeo SJ, Lo NN. Stress fracture of the medial tibial plateau after minimally invasive unicompartmental knee arthroplasty: a report of 2 cases. *J Arthroplasty* 2003; **18**: 801–3.

7. Sloper PJ, Hing CB, Donell ST, Glasgow MM. Intra-operative tibial plateau fracture during unicompartmental knee replacement: a case report. *Knee* 2003; **10**: 367–9.

8. Berger RA, Meneghini RM, Jacobs JJ, Sheinkop MB, Della Valle CJ, Rosenberg AG, Galante JO. Results of unicompartmental knee arthroplasty at a minimum of ten years of follow-up. *J Bone Joint Surg [Am]* 2005; **87-A**: 999–1006.

9. Goodfellow JW, O'Connor JJ, Shrive NG. Endoprosthetic knee joint devices. Br Patent 1534263, 1974.

10. Price AJ. Medial meniscal bearing unicompartmental arthroplasty: wear, mechanics and clinical outcome. DPhil Thesis, University of Oxford, 2003.

11. Jeer PJ, Keene GC, Gill P. Unicompartmental knee arthroplasty: an intermediate report of survivorship after the introduction of a new system with analysis of failures. *Knee* 2004; **11**: 369–74.

12. Dejour H, Dejour D, Habi S. Prothese Unicompartimentale du Genou. *Cah Enseign SOFCOT* 1998; **65**: 156–9.

13. Price AJ, Waite JC, Svard U. Long-term clinical results of the medial Oxford unicompartmental knee arthroplasty. *Clin Orthop* 2005; **435**: 171–80.

14. Psychoyios V, Crawford RW, O'Connor JJ, Murray DW. Wear of congruent meniscal bearings in unicompartmental knee arthroplasty: a retrieval study of 16 specimens. *J Bone Joint Surg [Br]* 1998; **80-B**: 976–82.

15. Vorlat P, Putzeys G, Cottenie D, Van Isacker T, Pouliart N, Handelberg F, Casteleyn PP, Gheysen F, Verdonk R. The Oxford unicompartmental knee prosthesis: an independent 10-year survival analysis. *Knee Surg Sports Traumatol Arthrosc* 2006 Jan; **14**: 40–5.

Appendix
Mathematical models of the knee

Introduction

Mathematical models make it possible to calculate quantities which are difficult or impossible to measure and provide insights which are not obtained from experiment alone. They are a necessary adjunct to the experimental method, but are not a common feature of biological or clinical research. A model is based on a series of assumptions or hypotheses about the way a physical system works. It is validated by comparing its predictions with independent experimental measurement. Reasonable validation then gives confidence in the assumptions on which the model is based and in the predictions of quantities which cannot be measured. The purpose in presenting our models here is to explain the differences between unloaded and loaded motion described in Chapter 1.

Many mathematical models of the natural knee [1–3] and of knee replacement have been proposed [4–6]. They have usually modelled the movement of the joint under load. We have found it easier to model the mobility of the knee in the absence of load, then the stability of the knee under load but in the absence of movement, and then to combine both to study activity, i.e. movement under load.

Three-dimensional model of knee mobility

The model (Fig. A1) explains the coupling of axial rotation to flexion and, more generally, how the joint achieves a range of unresisted passive mobility [7]. The model was formulated using the assumptions that the articular surfaces medially and laterally remain continuously in contact without interpenetration during passive flexion and that single fibres within each of the two cruciates and the MCL remain isometric. These five constraints to motion, when acting together, reduce the six possible degrees of freedom of the bones to one, so that axial rotation is coupled to flexion. The calculated coupling of axial rotation to flexion required to satisfy these assumptions agrees well with the measurements (Fig. A2).

Pictures of the model in extension and at 45° and 90° flexion (Fig. A1) show that during flexion the articular surfaces of the femur roll and slide on the surfaces of the tibia while the femur rotates externally on the tibia. The three isometric ligament fibres rotate about their insertions into the tibia. The sliding and rolling of the surfaces and the rotation of the ligament fibres are accomplished without tissue deformation and therefore without generating resistance to motion.

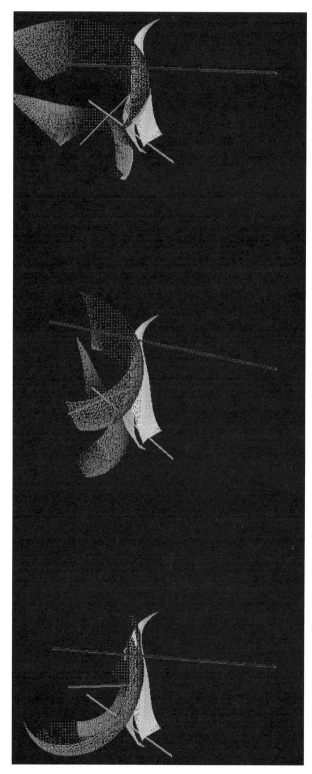

Figure A1 Three-dimensional model of knee mobility at extension, 45° flexion, and 90° flexion. The brown shells are the surfaces of the model femoral condyles, the yellow shells are the surfaces of the tibial plateaux, and the red, green, and blue lines are the isometric fibres of the ACL, PCL, and MCL, respectively.

An animation of the model is presented on the DVD Track 1 accompanying this book and demonstrates how the surfaces of the bones move on each other. The axial rotation of the surfaces of the femoral condyles can best be appreciated by watching the movements of their posterior edges.

The predictions of the model are sensitive to the choice of its parameters: (1) the shapes of the articular surfaces and (2) the positions of the points of origin and insertion of the isometric ligament fibres. If spherical femoral condyles and flat tibial surfaces are chosen, the result is greater anteroposterior movement of the contact points on the tibia in both compartments and larger values of coupled external femoral rotation. The model also demonstrates the important role of the MCL, and the absence of a role for the LCL, in guiding passive motion. If the model MCL is placed on the lateral rather than the medial side, obligatory internal rather than external rotation of the femur occurs during flexion, a result that is unlikely to be deduced except by modelling.

Two-dimensional model of the knee: the four-bar linkage

Mobility

The rolling and sliding movements of the femur on the tibia are more clearly seen in the simpler two-dimensional four-bar linkage model of Figure A3 (animated on the DVD Track 2) [8–11]. The figure shows the femur flexing on a fixed tibia with lines representing the extensor and flexor muscles. The distal surface of the femur has separate curves representing (1) the sulcus of the trochlea, anteriorly, in contact with the patella, and (2) the distal and posterior facets of the condyle in contact with the tibia. The model tibial articular surface is flat, a two-dimensional compromise between the slightly concave medial and slightly convex lateral plateaus of the human knee. Lines representing the isometric fibres of the two cruciates, rotating about their insertions on the tibia, and lines joining their attachments on the two bones form a crossed four-bar linkage [12]. The two-dimensional model separates the kinematics of the joint in the sagittal plane from the effects of coupled axial rotation.

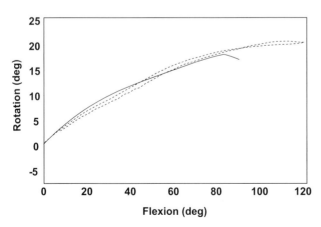

Figure A2 External rotation of the femur plotted against flexion angle. The solid line calculated from the three-dimensional model of mobility (Fig. A1) matches well the experimental curves of Fig. 1.16 (dotted lines).

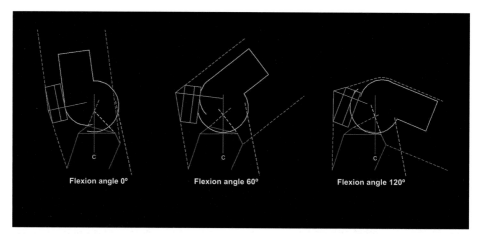

Figure A3 Two-dimensional four-bar linkage model of the knee in which isometric fibres in the ACL (dashed) and PCL (dashed white) guide the rolling and sliding movements of the femur on the tibia during passive flexion–extension. The point of contact C between the articular surfaces of the bones lies on the perpendicular to the tibial plateau through the intersection of the ligament fibres. Muscle tendons are shown as single lines. The rectangular model of the patella is held between the quadriceps and patellar tendons (dashed green). The hamstrings tendon and the gastrocnemius tendon are shown by pink and blue dashed lines, respectively.

The flexion axis of the joint passes through the point of intersection of the isometric ligament fibres (the 'instant centre' of the linkage) and moves backwards relative to the tibia during flexion, and forwards during extension. The point of contact between the femoral condyle and the flat tibial surface of the model always lies on the perpendicular to the tibial plateau through the flexion axis and therefore also moves backwards on the tibia during flexion and forwards during extension (as indicated by the vertical lines marked C in Fig. A3). The femur rolls as well as slides on the tibia; it rolls backwards (while sliding forwards) during flexion, and rolls forwards (while sliding backwards) during extension. The calculated value of the slip ratio (movement of the contact point on the tibia divided by its movement on the femur) varies between 0.2 and 0.4, similar to the range of values estimated by Feikes [13] for the intact cadaver knee. The model contact point moves backwards 11 mm over 120° flexion, similar to the mean value of its movement (10 mm) in human knees [13].

Therefore the model describes the average behaviour of the two compartments without axial rotation. The isometric ligament fibres keep the articular surfaces continuously in contact, and the articular surfaces keep the ligament fibres just tight. Unresisted passive flexion and extension can occur without tissue deformation because the isometric fibres rotate about their insertions on the bones without stretching, and the articular surfaces roll and slide on each other without indentation.

The directions of the model ligaments, the lengths of the lever arms of the flexor and extensor muscles, and their variation with flexion angle agree well with measurements on cadaver human knee specimens made by Hertzog and Read [14].

Ligament kinematics

The architecture of the ACL and PCL ligament arrays has been described by Friederich *et al.* [15] and Mommersteeg *et al.* [16], and the model's cruciate ligaments (Fig. A4) are based on those studies. The attachment areas are shown as straight lines, with a definite arrangement between the point of origin of an individual fibre and its point of insertion. Tight fibres are shown as straight lines, and slack fibres are shown buckled.

The fibres of the model ACL are straight, almost parallel, just tight in extension, and attached to the femur along the line ab Fig. A4(a). The PCL is modelled as two bundles of fibres attached to the femur along the lines ca and ab, with the anterior bundle being slack and the posterior bundle just tight in extension (Fig. A4(d)). Five representative fibres are drawn in the ACL and in each bundle of the PCL, but the mathematics assumes a continuous distribution of fibres along each attachment line. The most anterior ACL fibre ay and the most anterior of the PCL posterior bundle ay are the isometric fibres of Figure A3, and the relative motion of the bones is the same in both figures.

During flexion of the joint to 120°, the femoral attachment areas of both ligaments rotate through 120° relative to the tibia, appearing to pivot about the insertions of the

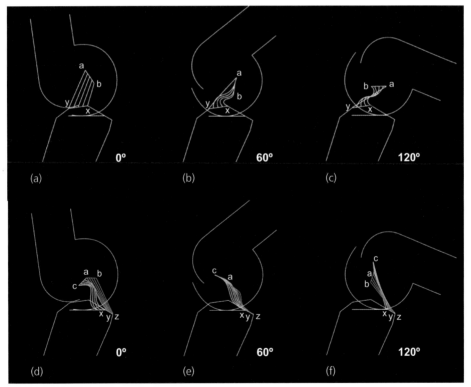

Figure A4 Model knee with arrays of fibres representing the ACL and two bundles of the PCL, attached to the femur along ab and cab respectively. (At 60°, the attachment point b of the PCL lies under the fibres and has not been identified.)

isometric fibres. As a result, the ligaments change their shapes. In both ligaments, fibres originating along the attachment line ab are more or less parallel in extension but are crossed on each other at 120°. Cross-over occurs when the attachment line ab lies along the isometric fibre ay. This occurs at about 70° flexion for the ACL and 60° flexion for the posterior fibres of the PCL (see DVD Track 3).

Fibres passing behind the intersection of the isometric fibres slacken during flexion and tighten during extension. Fibres passing in front of the intersection of the isometric fibres tighten during flexion and slacken during extension. Prior to cross-over, points of origin and insertion in the ACL and in the posterior bundle of the PCL approach each other during flexion, and fibres slacken. After cross-over, these points depart from each other and fibres tighten. The anterior fibres of the model PCL pass in front of the intersection of the isometric fibres and tighten during flexion as its femoral attachment area AC rotates away from the tibia. They are just tight and straight at 120°. Thus, most ligament fibres are slack in most positions of the unloaded joint. No fibres are stretched.

The changes in shape of the model ACL are very similar to those reported in the cadaver human knee using Röntgen stereometric analysis [17] and to the sketches of Friederich *et al.* [18] and Girgis *et al.* [19]. The shape changes of the model PCL are similar to the sketches of Brantigan and Voschell [20], and the patterns of fibre slackening and tightening predicted by the model are quantitatively similar to those measured in cadaver knees [21–25]. These comparisons with experiment serve to validate the model and the assumptions on which it is based.

The DVD Track 4 contains an animation of a knee model with arrays of fibres representing all four principal ligaments, including the two cruciates of Figure A4. Many observers agree that all fibres within the LCL become slack once flexion begins [26–29]. This is because the fibres always lie behind the flexion axis of the joint.

The behaviour of the model MCL demonstrates one of the deficiencies of a two-dimensional model. The fibres of that ligament cover the intersection of the two isometric cruciate fibres so that the flexion axis of the joint passes through the ligament. As a result, the most anterior of the superficial fibres of the model MCL stretch during passive flexion. However, the two-dimensional model does not account for obligatory axial rotation. The associated forward movement of the femoral attachment area of the MCL relative to the tibia, as seen in the three-dimensional model in Figure A1 (and in the animation on the DVD Track 1), slackens these stretched fibres and allows unresisted flexion. This feature of the two-dimensional model prompted the development of the three-dimensional model and the incorporation of an isometric MCL fibre in addition to the cruciates.

Discussion

The rolling of the femur on the tibia during passive flexion–extension is required to minimize ligament strain in the unloaded knee and allow unresisted passive movement. Predictions of the mathematical models of passive motion compare well with measurements made on cadaver specimens in our own and other laboratories, validating the principal assumptions underlying the models, i.e. that the human knee behaves as a mechanism during passive motion, guided by the articular surfaces in contact and by isometric fibres within the cruciates and the MCL. Every implantation of an Oxford prosthesis which succeeds in matching the 90° flexion gap to the 20° flexion gap when the bone surfaces are distracted by feeler gauges is evidence of ligament isometricity. The slack model LCL in the flexed knee is believed to explain the high rate of bearing dislocation in lateral OUKA (see Chapter 3).

These concepts have recently been challenged by Freeman [30], without confronting the many experimental validations of the models but on the grounds that the PCL is (apparently) slack in flexion, an argument advanced by Strasser in 1917 [31] in a criticism of the first description of the four-bar linkage model given by Zuppinger in 1904 [32]. All fibres of a ligament cannot be isometric unless they all originate on or pass through the flexion axis of the joint. Slackness of most fibres does not preclude the isometry of some. The isometric fibres within the PCL lie within the body of the ligament and are difficult to observe visually. Nonetheless, the shapes of the model ligament in extension and flexion shown in Figure A4 are very similar to those shown in Section 8 of Freeman's booklet [30], and are consequences of the isometricity of some fibres, not an argument against it. The changes of fibre length in the PCL predicted by the model are very similar to those described by Garg and Walker [33] and by Covey *et al.* [25]. Freeman also shows how the PCL is readily deflected sideways by a transverse force. But even a very tight rope, like a bowstring, offers little resistance to transverse motion of a point in the middle of its span. A better demonstration of the function of the PCL is to show how its slack fibres are systematically recruited to resist backward movement of the tibia relative to the femur when the knee is appropriately loaded.

Stability of the loaded joint

Figure A5 shows how the model ACL responds when the tibia is moved backwards and forwards relative to the femur (as in a drawer test) at a fixed flexion angle [34,35]. With the unloaded knee flexed to 50°, all but the anterior fibres of the ACL are slack (Fig. A5(b)). When the tibia is pushed backwards 5 mm from the neutral position, the anterior fibre slackens and all other fibres slacken further (Fig. A5(a)). When the tibia is

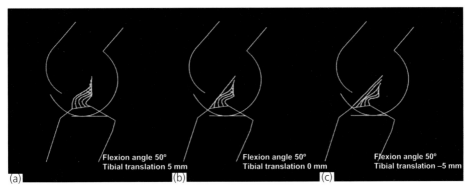

Flexion angle 50°
Tibial translation 5 mm
(a)

Flexion angle 50°
Tibial translation 0 mm
(b)

Flexion angle 50°
Tibial translation –5 mm
(c)

Figure A5 Fibres of the model ACL, with the knee at 50° flexion, (a) slacken and (c) tighten when the tibia is pulled backward and forward from the neutral unloaded position (b).

pulled forwards 5 mm from its neutral position, ACL fibres are progressively tightened and stretched to bear load (Fig. A5(c)). A 5 mm anterior translation tightens and stretches about half the model ACL (see DVD Track 5).

Figure A6 (and the DVD Track 6) show similar diagrams of the model knee with all four ligaments modelled as arrays of fibres. Posterior translation of the tibia (Fig A6(a)) tightens the PCL and the LCL, and slackens the ACL and the MCL. Anterior translation (Fig A6(c)) tightens the ACL and the MCL, and slackens the PCL and the LCL. The ligaments offer increasing resistance to anteroposterior displacement from the neutral position (Fig. A6(b)) as more and more fibres are recruited to bear load, giving the knee its characteristic laxity. The laxity allowed by ligament strain is further increased by indentation of the articular surfaces under load [36]. The calculation of the anteroposterior laxity of the model joint under a drawer force of 67 N by Huss *et al.* [36] agrees well with measurements made by Grood and Noyes [37], providing a validation of the model.

Discussion

The laxity allowed by stretching of the ligaments should be recovered after unconstrained unicompartmental arthroplasty which retains all the ligaments and restores them to their natural tensions. The contribution to laxity attributed to deformation of the surfaces will be lost when they are replaced by more rigid prosthetic components. However, the contribution of surface deformation in the intact joint is relatively small.

Mathematical model of OUKA

A two-dimensional mathematical model of OUKA created by Imran [38] explains the observed differences between passive and active flexion referred to in Chapter 1.

The sequence of images in Figure A7 represents passive motion in the absence of load. Those in Figure A8 model a drawer test, with the bones at a fixed flexion angle and moved anteroposteriorly relative to each other by an external force against the resistance of the ligaments.

The model of passive motion (Fig. A7) finds the position of the femur on the tibia which minimizes ligament strain. The anteroposterior position of the femur on the tibia was adjusted mathematically, as in Figure A8(b), until both cruciate ligaments had just fully slackened, with zero force in each. This condition requires rollback of the femur on the tibia and consequently, posterior translation of the meniscal bearing during flexion (see DVD Track 7).

The patterns of fibre strain in Figure A7 are very similar to those in Figure A4 which were based on the assumed presence of the two isometric fibres of Figure A3. Therefore the model in Figure A7 predicts rather than assumes the presence of isometric fibres. It is emphasized that the only inputs to the model were the geometry of the arrays of fibres, the positions of the prosthetic components, the femoral trochlea, and the tibial tubercle relative to the ligament attachment areas, the length of the patellar tendon, and the shape of the model patella. The positions of the bones relative to each other were then calculated using the laws of geometry and mechanics. The model of passive mobility (Fig. A7) predicts passive bearing movements very similar to those observed fluoroscopically (Fig. 1.19).

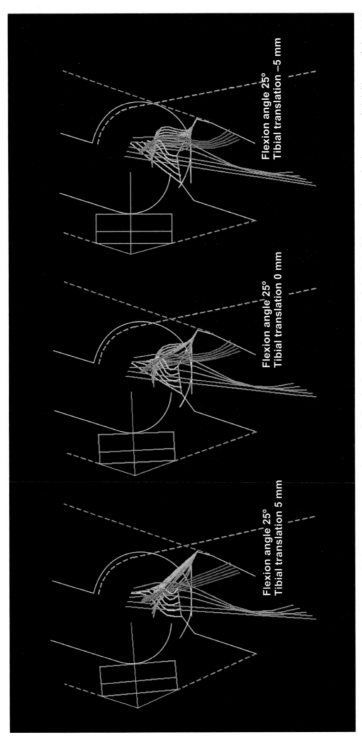

Figure A6 Model knee with arrays of fibres representing the ACL (yellow), the two bundles of the PCL (blue and green), the superficial fibres of the MCL (purple), and the LCL (red). Fibres within the PCL and LCL tighten and those within the ACL and MCL slacken when the tibia is pushed backwards (a) from the neutral position (b), and vice versa when the tibia is pulled forward (c) from the neutral position.

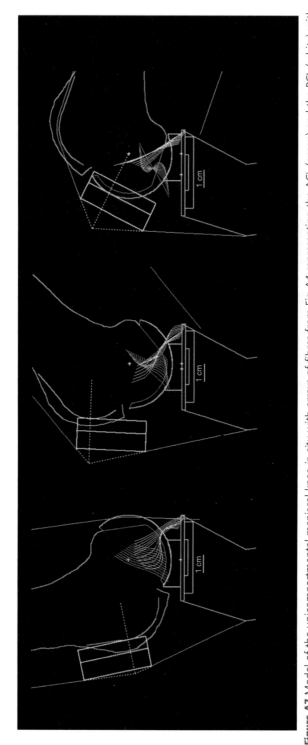

Figure A7 Model of the unicompartmental meniscal knee *in situ* with arrays of fibres from Fig A4 representing the ACL (green) and the PCL (white) with the extensor mechanism and hamstrings tendon of Figure A3. At each flexion angle, the position of the femur on the tibia was that which produced zero force in each cruciate ligament.

Model of the leg-lift exercise

Comparison of Figures A7 and A8 shows that the anteroposterior movements of the meniscal bearing on the tibia required to tighten slack ligaments are similar in magnitude to those which occur during passive movements. These two effects are superimposed in activity and can augment or cancel each other. Figure A9 shows a model of leg-lift with the femur horizontal and the weight of the leg balanced by tension forces in the patellar and quadriceps tendons. In extension, the patellar tendon pulls the tibia upwards, a movement resisted by tension in the ACL (and MCL). All fibres of the ACL are shown stretched tight. The stretch of the ligament allows the femur (and the bearing) to move backwards on the tibial plateau relative to their positions in the unloaded joint. As the knee bends and the leg falls, the forces in the ACL (and MCL) diminish. At 57° (Fig. A9(b)), only the most anterior fibre of the ACL is just tight and the bearing lies close to its corresponding position in the unloaded joint. With further flexion, the PCL begins to tighten and stretch and the ACL goes completely slack, allowing the femur to move forward relative to its position in the unloaded joint. Therefore the total excursion of the bearing on the tibia is much reduced compared with passive motion, because of the stretching of the ligaments. While this two-dimensional model does not account for axial rotation and does not therefore predict exactly the observed pattern of bearing movement during active extension–flexion (Fig. 1.19), it demonstrates the effects of ligament strain and explains the differences between active and passive motion observed fluoroscopically.

In the unloaded state the meniscal bearing moves to that position which minimizes ligament strain, requiring rollback of the femur on the tibia. Under load, the bearing moves to the position required to balance ligament and muscle force components parallel to the tibial plateau. These criteria are different and the movements of the bearings are also different. This analysis validates the assertion we made in 1978 that 'the components [of a knee prosthesis] should allow and should not resist the movements demanded by the soft tissues' [39]. This criterion can also be satisfied by unconstrained two-component designs but at the expense of excessive wear. The fully congruent meniscal bearing meets the criteria of both minimum wear and minimum constraint.

Ligament mechanics

The patterns of ligament strain during passive motion can be modelled with or without the assumption of isometry, with similar results. Because of these isometric fibres, the width of the gap between the femoral and tibial components of the prosthesis in the medial component remains constant over the range of passive flexion and can be filled with a rigid meniscal bearing of the appropriate thickness.

The patellofemoral joint

The model patella used in our two-dimensional models [10] is shown as a rectangle in Figures A3, A6, A9, and A10 with two straight-line articular surfaces parallel to its anterior surface. In addition to a circle defining the sulcus of the trochlea, Figures A7–A10 contain a more anterior curve outlining the flanges of the trochlea.

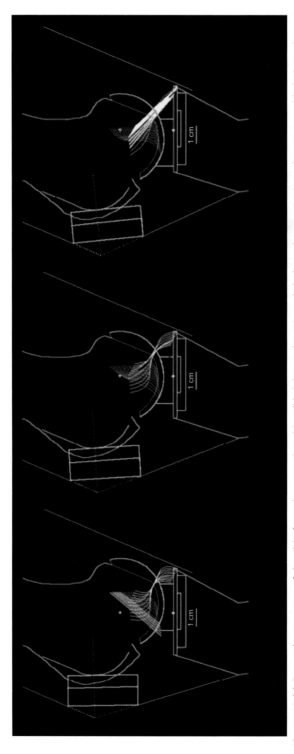

Figure A8 (a) Forward movement of the tibia from the neutral position (b) tightens the ACL and slackens the PCL. Backward movement (c) slackens the ACL and tightens the PCL (see DVD Track 8).

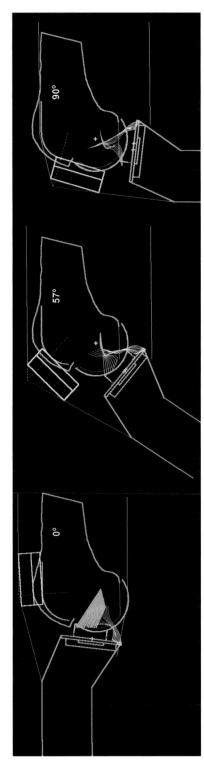

Figure A9 Model of active flexion–extension when the weight of the leg is balanced by tension in the patellar tendon. In extension (a), the tibia is pulled anteriorly relative to the femur, the ACL is stretched, and the PCL is slack. At 57°, all fibres of both ligaments are just slack. At 90°, the PCL has begun to tighten. The excursion of the meniscal bearing on the tibia is reduced compared with passive flexion (Fig. A7) (see DVD Track 9).

The most posterior surface of the model patella, representing the median ridge of the human patella, makes contact with the femoral trochlea at extension and over most of the flexion range. The more anterior surface represents the medial and lateral facets of the patella. Patellofemoral contact occurs near the distal pole of the patella in extension (Figs. A3(a) and A7(a)), and moves proximally (Figs. A3(b) and A7(b)) with increasing flexion. Eventually, contact moves onto the medial and lateral facets of the patella, and onto the femoral condyle (Fig. A3(c)) or the femoral component (Fig. A7(c)). The median ridge (the anterior articular surface) then passes into the intercondylar notch and lies proximal to the articular surface of the femur.

The predicted movement of the contact area on the model patella is very similar to that observed in the human knee (see Fig. 2.19) [40]. The patella rolls proximally as it slides distally on the femur during knee flexion, ensuring that the line of action of the patellofemoral contact force always passes through the intersection of the patellar and quadriceps tendons, a condition necessary for mechanical equilibrium of the patella [10].

A number of the predictions of patellofemoral behaviour from this model agree well with independent measurements [41]. The quadriceps tendon is shown as a line extending proximally from the proximal pole of the model patella (Figs. A3, A6, A7–A10). At

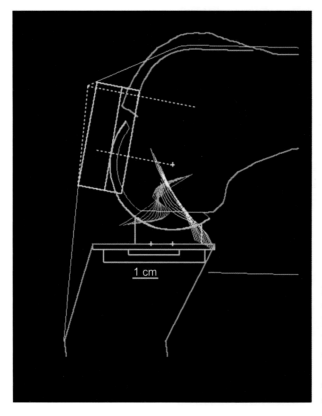

Figure A10 Model knee at 99° flexion when patellar contact is about to transfer from the trochlea to the femoral component. The perpendiculars to the surfaces of the patella at the two contact points are parallel.

high flexion angles (>85°), it wraps around the trochlea to form the tendofemoral joint, as described by Bishop and Denham [42]. The angle between the quadriceps and the patellar tendons, called the patella mechanism angle, diminishes with increasing knee flexion. The variation of this angle as calculated from the model agrees well with measurements by Buff *et al.* [43]. The angles between each of the tendons and the line of action of the patellofemoral force are not equal, and as a result the tension forces in the two tendons are not equal [44]. The variation of the ratio of the tendon forces with flexion angle calculated from the model agrees well with measurements [42,43,45,46].

The instant of transition from trochlear contact to condylar contact is shown in Figure A10, with the model knee drawn at 99° flexion. Contact is about to move from the trochlea onto the femoral component. The patella is held anteriorly on the trochlea until its medial and lateral facets overlie the femoral component. The anterior edge of the femoral component is bypassed and is never in contact with the patella, so that there is no danger of the type of impingement described by Hernigou and Deschamps [47] as a common complication of fixed-bearing polycentric unicompartmental arthroplasties.

The models of the intact and replaced joints both demonstrate changes in PTA with flexion similar to those observed in living patients (Fig. 1.18) with complete restoration of function. This may be a reason why revision of an OUKA for patellar problems is rare.

Conclusion

Experimental and mathematical studies of the mobility and stability of the normal knee show that each requires interaction between the articular surfaces and the ligaments.

The joint achieves its mobility because the surfaces can roll and slide on each other while the ligaments rotate about their origins and insertions on the bones. The articular surfaces keep some fibres of the ligaments just tight over the range of movement, while the ligaments keep the surfaces just in contact. These interactions require no tissue deformation and give the joint its range of unresisted motion, leading to the coupling of axial rotation to flexion angle and to femoral rollback.

The joint achieves its stability because the articular surfaces resist indentation under compressive forces and the ligaments resist elongation under tensile forces. As load increases, the indentations and elongations continue and the contact areas adjust until the ligament forces balance the applied loads and muscle forces. This mechanism gives the joint its characteristic laxity, requiring rapidly increasing applied loads to move the bones from their passive positions.

In activity, motion occurs under load and the mechanisms which control mobility and stability are combined.

All these features of natural mobility and stability can be restored to a satisfactory extent by retaining all ligaments and implanting fully unconstrained prosthetic components which allow but do not resist the movements required by the soft tissues. Polyethylene wear can be minimized by the use of fully conforming mobile meniscal bearings. Exact reproduction of the shapes of the natural articular surfaces is not required. The balance between restoration of function and resistance to wear is achieved by the use of spherical and flat articular surfaces on the metal components with an interposed fully conforming meniscal bearing.

References

1. Crowninshield R, Pope MH, Johnson R, Miller R. The impedance of the human knee. *J Biomech* 1976; **9**: 529–35.

2. Andriacchi TP, Mikosz RP, Hampton SJ, Galante JO. Model studies of the stiffness characteristics of the human knee joint. *J Biomech* 1983; **16**: 23–9.

3. Blankevoort L, Huiskes R. Validation of a three-dimensional model of the knee. *J Biomech* 1996; **29**: 955–61.

4. Sathasivam S, Walker PS. Optimization of the bearing surface geometry of total knees. *J Biomech* 1994; **27**: 255–64.

5. Sathasivam S, Walker PS. A computer model with surface friction for the prediction of total knee kinematics. *J Biomech* 1997; **30**: 177–84.

6. Sathasivam S, Walker PS. Computer model to predict subsurface damage in tibial inserts of total knees. *J Orthop Res* 1998; **16**: 564–71.

7. Wilson DR, Feikes JD, O'Connor JJ. Ligaments and articular contact guide passive knee flexion. *J Biomech* 1998; **31**: 1127–36.

8. O'Connor JJ, Shercliff TL, Biden E, Goodfellow JW. The geometry of the knee in the sagittal plane. *J Engng Med, Proc Inst Mech Eng [H]* 1989; **203**: 223–33.

9. Zavatsky AB, O'Connor JJ. A model of human knee ligaments in the sagittal plane. Part 1: Response to passive flexion. *J Engng Med, Proc Inst Mech Eng [H]* 1992; **206**: 125–34.

10. Gill HS, O'Connor JJ. Biarticulating two-dimensional computer model of the human patellofemoral joint. *Clin Biomech* 1996; **11**: 81–89.

11. Lu T-W, O'Connor JJ. Lines of action and moment arms of the major force-bearing structures crossing the human knee joint: comparison between theory and experiment. *J Anat* 1996; **189**: 575–85.

12. Hall AS. *Kinematics and Linkage Design*. Englewood Cliffs, NJ: Prentice-Hall, 1961.

13. Feikes JD. The mobility and stability of the human knee joint. DPhil Thesis, University of Oxford, 1999.

14. Herzog W, Read LJ. Lines of action and moment arms of the major force-carrying structures crossing the human knee joint. *J Anat* 1993; **182**: 213–30.

15. Friederich NF, Muller W, O'Brien WR. [Clinical application of biomechanic and functional anatomical findings of the knee joint]. *Orthopäde* 1992; **21**: 41–50.

16. Mommersteeg TJ, Blankevoort L, Huiskes R, Kooloos JG, Kauer JM, Hendriks JC. The effect of variable relative insertion orientation of human knee bone–ligament–bone complexes on the tensile stiffness. *J Biomech* 1995; **28**: 745–52.

17. van Dijk R, Huiskes R, Selvik G. Roentgen stereophotogrammetric methods for the evaluation of the three dimensional kinematic behavior and cruciate ligament length patterns of the human knee. *J Biomech* 1979; **12**: 727–31.

18. Friederich NF, O'Brien WR. Anterior cruciate ligament graft tensioning versus knee stability. *Knee Surg Sports Traumatol Arthrosc* 1998; **6**(Suppl 1): S38–42.

19. Girgis FG, Marshall JL, Monajem A. The cruciate ligaments of the knee joint. Anatomical, functional and experimental analysis. *Clin Orthop* 1975; **106**: 216–31.

20. Brantigan OC, Voshell AF. The mechanics of the ligaments and menisci of the knee joint. *J Bone Joint Surg [Am]* 1941; **23-A**: 44–66.

21. Sidles JA, Larson RV, Garbini JL, Downey DJ, Matsen FAI. Ligament length relationships in the moving knee. *J Orthop Res* 1988; **6**: 593–610.

22. Sapega AA, Moyer MA, Schneck C, Komalahiranya N. Testing for isometry during reconstruction of the anterior cruciate ligament. *J Bone Joint Surg [Am]* 1990; **72-A**: 259–67.

23. Garg A, Walker PS. Prediction of total knee motion using a three-dimensional computer- graphics model. *J Biomech* 1990; **23**: 45–58.

24. Amis AA, Dawkins GPC. Functional anatomy of the anterior cruciate ligament: fibre bundle actions related to ligament replacements and injuries. *J Bone Joint Surg [Br]* 1991; **73-B**: 260–7.

25. Covey DC, Sapega AA, Sherman GM, Torg JS. Testing for 'isometry' during posterior cruciate ligament reconstruction. *Trans Orthop Res Soc*; 1992; **17**; 665.

26. Meister BR, Michael SP, Moyer RA, Kelly JD, Schneck CD. Anatomy and kinematics of the lateral collateral ligament of the knee. *Am J Sports Med* 2000; **28**: 869–78.

27. Wang C, Walker PS. The effects of flexion and rotation on the length patterns of the ligaments of the knee. *J Biomech* 1973; **6**: 587–96.

28. Rovick JS, Reuben JD, Schrager RJ, Walker PS. Relation between knee motion and ligament length patterns. *Clin Biomech* 1991; **6**: 213–20.

29. Robinson B. Dislocation in mobile bearing lateral unicompartmental arthroplasty. DPhil Thesis, University of Oxford, 2002.

30. Freeman MAR. *Tibiofemoral Movement*. London: British Editorial Society of Bone and Joint Surgery, 2001.

31. Strasser H. *Lehrbuch der Muskel und Gelenkmechanik. III Band: Die untere Extremitart*. Berlin: Springer-Verlag, 1917.

32. Zuppinger H. *Die Active Flexion im Umbelasteten Kniegelenk*. Weisbaden: Bergmann, 1904.

33. Garg A, Walker PS. The effect of the interface on the bone stresses beneath tibial components. *J Biomech* 1986; **19**: 957–67.

34. Zavatsky AB, O'Connor JJ. A model of human knee ligaments in the sagittal plane. Part 2: Fibre recruitment under load. *J Engng Med, Proc Inst Mech Eng [H]* 1992; **206**: 135–45.

35. Lu TW, O'Connor JJ. Fibre recruitment and shape changes of knee ligaments during motion: as revealed by a computer graphics-based model. *J Engng Med, Proc Inst Mech Eng [H]* 1996; **210**: 71–9.

36. Huss RA, Holstein H, O'Connor JJ. The effect of cartilage deformation on the laxity of the knee joint. *J Engng Med, Proc Inst Mech Eng [H]* 1999; **213**: 19–32.

37. Grood ES, Noyes FR. Diagnosis of knee ligament injuries: biomechanical precepts. In: Feagin JA Jr (ed) *The Crucial Ligaments: Diagnosis and Treatment of Ligamentous Injuries about the Knee*. New York: Churchill Livingstone, 1988; 245–85.

38. Imran A. Mechanics of the ligament deficient knee. DPhil Thesis, University of Oxford, 1999.

39. Goodfellow J, O'Connor J. The mechanics of the knee and prosthesis design. *J Bone Joint Surg [Br]* 1978; **60-B**: 358–69.

40. Goodfellow J, Hungerford DS, Zindel M. Patello-femoral joint mechanics and pathology. 1: Functional anatomy of the patello-femoral joint. *J Bone Joint Surg [Br]* 1976; **58-B**: 287–90.

41. O'Connor J, Shercliff T, FitzPatrick D. Mechanics of the knee. In: Daniel D, Akeson W, O'Connor J (ed) *Ligaments: Structure, Function, Injury and Repair*. New York: Raven Press, 1990.

42. Bishop R, Denham R. A note on the ratio between tensions in the quadriceps tendon and infrapatellar ligament. *Eng Med* 1977: **6**; 53–4.

43. Buff HU, Jones LC, Hungerford DS. Experimental determination of forces transmitted through the patello-femoral joint. *J Biomech* 1988; **21**: 17–23.

44. Maquet P. *Biomechanics of the Knee*. Berlin: Springer-Verlag, 1976.

45. Ellis MI, Seedhom BB, Wright V. Forces in the knee joint whilst rising from a seated position. *J Biomed Eng* 1984; **6**: 113–20.

46. Huberti HH, Hayes WC, Stone JL, Shybut GT. Force ratios in the quadriceps tendon and ligamentum patellae. *J Orthop Res* 1984; **2**: 49–54.

47. Hernigou P, Deschamps G. Patellar impingement following unicompartmental arthroplasty. *J Bone Joint Surg [Am]* 2002; **84-A**: 1132–7.

Index